INTERMITTENT FASTING FOR WOMEN OVER 50

The Ultimate Guide to Detox and Rejuvenate your Body, Reset Metabolism and Accelerate Weight Loss with Intermittent Fasting Diet

Emily Jackson

© Copyright 2021 - All rights reserved.

The content contained within this book may not be reproduced, duplicated or transmitted without direct written permission from the author or the publisher.

Under no circumstances will any blame or legal responsibility be held against the publisher, or author, for any damages, reparation, or monetary loss due to the information contained within this book. Either directly or indirectly.

Legal Notice:

This book is copyright protected. This book is only for personal use. You cannot amend, distribute, sell, use, quote or paraphrase any part, or the content within this book, without the consent of the author or publisher.

Disclaimer Notice:

Please note the information contained within this document is for educational and entertainment purposes only. All effort has been executed to present accurate, up to date, and reliable, complete information. No warranties of any kind are declared or implied. Readers acknowledge that the author is not engaging in the rendering of legal, financial, medical or professional advice. The content within this book has been derived from various sources. Please consult a licensed professional before attempting any techniques outlined in this book.

By reading this document, the reader agrees that under no circumstances is the author responsible for any losses, direct or indirect, which are incurred as a result of the use of information contained within this document, including, but not limited to, errors, omissions, or inaccuracies.

Table of Contents

Introduction

Females over 50 can be prone to a range of medical issues, including osteoporosis, hormone imbalances, urinary tract infections, thyroid disorders, and more. These conditions can make it more difficult for women over 50 to eat regular meals and adhere to healthy eating patterns. Osteoporosis is a medical condition that occurs when the bones become fragile and weak due to low diet, lack of exercise, or other lifestyle factors.

Osteoporosis has been linked to depression, insomnia, and memory loss. It can also increase the risk of fracture due to falls or accidents. Women who experience fractures caused by osteoporosis are more likely to have complications such as infection or pain.

Intermittent fasting for women over 50 is a specialized form of intermittent fasting that can be done without feeling like you are depriving your body of food. Unlike other intermittent fasting forms, intermittent fasting for women over 50 will not limit your intake of calories or nutrients. It promotes healthy eating habits and encourages the use of whole foods in their natural state. It also has the added benefit of regulating your menstrual cycle, reducing appetite, and promoting positive feelings about your body.

The advantages of intermittent fasting for women over 50 are numerous: You will feel happier and healthier. You will have the energy to get through the day. You will have more time for self-care and enjoyment (think exercise, hobbies, socializing). Your blood pressure and insulin levels will be lower. Your eyesight and digestive health may improve because you won't be eating large quantities of food in a short timeframe. It may promote sleep. Women who follow an intermittent fasting schedule tend to have more sex than those who don't, so that alone should be a selling point!

Several studies have confirmed that intermittent fasting prevents obesity in both mice and humans. In mice, intermittent fasting led to a significant drop in body weight and improved cholesterol levels. A study conducted on 18 obese women showed that participants who practiced intermittent fasting experienced substantial weight loss without any calorie restriction. Another study on 16 overweight men showed substantial body fat decreases after adopting a 10/14-day fasting schedule.

In humans, intermittent fasting is beneficial for people suffering from anorexia because it reverses leptin resistance. This condition causes overeating and rapidly increasing fat deposition in the belly and thighs. Another study among obese children and adolescents showed that intermittent fasting helped lower their cholesterol levels and better glucose and insulin regulation. As this type of diet becomes more popular among older women seeking to lose weight but without resorting to calorie restriction, doctors are starting to talk about the benefits of alternating periods of fasting with eating during the day.

Intermittent fasting is a way of fasting that doesn't require you to stop eating completely. Instead, you cycle your fasting schedule to include more eating during some days than others. This helps you maintain your muscle and strength while you sleep away the calories stored during your fast.

The idea of intermittent fasting was popularized in the 1970s by Dr. Jason Fung in his book, The Obesity Code: Unlocking the Secrets of Weight Loss. Intermittent fasting is also known as time-restricted feeding (TRF) or alternate-day fasting (ADF).

Intermittent fasting works best for those who have an average body mass index (BMI). People who are overweight or obese should not use intermittent fasting because it can cause weight loss to be slower than usual.

CHAPTER 1:

Science of Intermittent Fasting

Understanding the science behind why Intermittent Fasting works will help you to feel confident and comfortable as you change your diet and lifestyle to accommodate this new regime. We will begin by answering the question, what is autophagy, before moving on to more specific aspects of this interesting cellular process in the body.

What Is Autophagy?

Autophagy is a process that happens within the human body that has been going on without our knowledge since the beginning of human existence. It is only recently that people have begun to harness this process to achieve desired positive results through changes in their diet, such as Intermittent Fasting. We will look at this topic in-depth throughout this book, but here we will begin by looking at what exactly autophagy is.

Autophagy, as a word, can be broken up into two individual parts. Each of these parts on its own is a separate Greek word—the word 'auto', which means self, and the word 'phagy,' which means the practice of eating. Putting these together gives you the practice of self-eating, which is essentially what autophagy is. This may sound a little intimidating. Still, it is a very natural process that our cells practice all the time without us being any the wiser. Autophagy is the body's way of cleaning itself out.

Essentially, the body has housekeepers that keep everything neat and tidy. Scientists who have been studying this for some time are now beginning to understand that there are ways to manipulate this process within your body to achieve weight loss, improved health, reduction of disease symptoms, and so on. This is what we will spend the rest of the book looking at, but first, we will dive into the science of autophagy a little more.

How Does Autophagy Work?

The process of autophagy involves small "hunter" particles that go around your body, looking for cells or cell components that are old and damaged. The hunter particles then take these cell components apart, getting rid of the damaged parts and saving the useful features to make new cells later. These hunter cells can also use helpful leftover pieces to create energy for the body.

Autophagy has been found to happen in all organisms that are multi-cellular, like animals and plants, in addition to humans. While the study of these larger organisms and how autophagy works in their cells is lesser-known, more studies are being done on humans and how diet changes can affect their body's autophagy.

The other function that autophagy serves is that it helps cells carry out their death when it is time for them to die. There are times when cells are programmed to die because of several different factors. Sometimes these cells need assistance in their death, and autophagy can help them with this or clean up after their death. The human body is all about life and death. These processes are continually going on without our knowledge to keep us healthy and in good form.

As I mentioned, the autophagy process has been going on inside us since the beginning of human existence. This process has been kept around inside our bodies because of the many benefits it can provide us with. It is also essential for our bodies' health, as being able to get rid of waste and damaged parts that are no longer useful to us is essential to our health. If we could not get rid of damaged or broken cells, these damaged particles would build up and eventually make us sick. Our bodies are incredibly efficient in everything that they do, and waste disposal is no different.

In more recent years, the study of autophagy has focused more heavily on diet and disease research. These studies are still in their early stages as it has been only a few years shy of sixty years since autophagy was discovered. This process was found in a lab by testing what happened when small organisms went without food for some time. These organisms were observed very closely under a microscope. It was found that their cells had this process of waste disposal and energy creation that was later named autophagy.

More about autophagy and its relation to energy production is being studied in recent years, as this topic is interesting to humans. Autophagy can use old cell parts and recycle them to create new energy that the organism (like the human or animal) can use to do its regular functions, like walking and breathing. Now, people are studying what happens when humans rely on this form of energy production instead of the energy they would get from ingesting food throughout the day. This is where autophagy and intermittent fasting come together. We will delve deeply into intermittent fasting and autophagy and how they work together to allow for things like weight loss or disease prevention.

What Does Autophagy Do?

Autophagy has many functions in the body. This section will look at some of the other autophagy functions and the body systems involved.

Autophagy is said to be the housekeeping function of the body. If you think of your body as your home, autophagy is the housekeeper you hire to take care of all of the waste and the recycling functions of your cells.

One of the housekeeping duties includes removing cell parts that were built wrongly or at the wrong time. Sometimes cells make mistakes, and these mistakes can cause proteins or other cell parts to be formed in error. When this happens, we need something within the cell to get rid of these so that they do not take up space or get in the way of other processes within the cell. Further, sometimes useful parts of the cell will become damaged, and then will need to be removed to make way for a new feature to take its place. These cell parts can include those that create DNA or those that create the proteins needed to make the DNA.

Another duty of autophagy is to protect the body from disease and pathogens. Pathogens are bacteria or viruses that can infect our cells and our bodies if they are not adequately defended. Autophagy works to kill the cells within our body infected by these pathogens to get rid of them before spreading. In this way, autophagy plays a part in our immune system. It acts as a supplement to our immune cells, whose sole function is to protect us from disease and infection invasions. Autophagy also functions to help the body's cells regulate themselves when there are stressors placed upon them. These stressors can be things like a lack of food for the cell or physical stresses placed on the cell. This regulation helps to maintain a standard cell environment despite factors that can change, like food availability. Autophagy can do things like break down cell parts for food to provide the cell with nutrients. Similar to its role in regulating the cells, autophagy also helps develop a growing fetus inside a woman's uterus. Autophagy occurs here to ensure that the embryo has enough nutrients and energy at all times for healthy development. In addition to this, it helps with growth in adults, and there is a balance of building new parts and breaking down old ones involved in the evolution of any organism.

Autophagy is more critical than we may even realize, as it plays a large role in the survival of the living organisms it acts within. It does this by being especially sensitive to the levels of nutrients and energy within a cell. When the nutrient levels lower, autophagy breaks down cell parts, creating nutrients, and if it weren't for this process, the cells would not maintain their ideal functioning environment. They may begin to make more mistakes and even lower their functional abilities altogether. So much goes on inside a cell that they need to work effectively at all times. Autophagy makes this possible, which is what makes it such an essential function.

Using Intermittent Fasting to Induce Autophagy

Autophagy functions in the following way. When a decrease in nutrients is noticed within a cell, this decrease in nutrients acts as a signal for the cell to create small pockets within a membrane (a thin barrier layer) called autophagosomes. These little pockets (autophagosomes) move through the cell and find debris and damaged particles floating around within the cell. The little pockets then consume this debris by absorbing it into its inner space. The waste is then enclosed in the membrane (the thin barrier layer) and is moved to a place in the cell called the Lysosome. A lysosome is a cell that acts as a center for degradation, breakdown, or disassembly. This part of the cell gets debris and damaged cell parts delivered to it by the autophagosomes. Once these damaged cell parts are offered, the lysosomes then break them down. By breaking them down, these parts can be recycled and used for energy.

The most common way to induce autophagy in a person is by way of starvation. This is not to say that a person must starve themselves, but they starve their cells of nutrition temporarily. This is why people turn to fasting to induce autophagy. Low nutrition levels within the cells are the most common way that autophagy is triggered, as it is a process that creates energy within the cell. By knowing this, scientists have concluded that by inducing starvation within the cells, one can intentionally upregulate autophagy in one body. Intermittent fasting involves periods of fasting, which then causes a state of hunger within the cells (merely meaning that there is no energy being consumed to use for life), and so it induces autophagy in the cells to make energy.

Other Ways to Induce Autophagy

Starvation

The most common way to induce autophagy in a person is by way of starvation. Autophagy is triggered by a decrease in nutrients within a cell. As I mentioned above, this decrease in nutrients acts as a signal within the cell to begin autophagy, precisely how Intermittent fasting works.

Aerobic Exercise

One other way to activate autophagy is through exercise. Aerobic exercise has been shown through studies to increase autophagy in the cells of the muscles, the heart, the brain, lungs, and the liver.

Sleep

Sleep is essential for autophagy. If you have ever gone a few days without proper, restful sleep, you know that you begin to feel a decline in your mental abilities rather quickly. This could be because of your brain's decreased autophagy functioning. The number of hours you are in bed does not matter if the sleep is not good quality. Quality sleep for the right number of hours is needed to maintain useful brain function and keep your brain's autophagy going.

Specific Foods

The consumption of specific foods has been shown to induce or promote autophagy. The added benefit is that not only do they trigger autophagy in the cells of your body, but these foods are also shown to have numerous other health benefits.

CHAPTER 2:

Why Intermittent Fasting

Over the age of 50, it is increasingly difficult for a woman to lose weight, and we are obsessed with those extra pounds that accumulate in areas where we do not want them, such as hips and love handles. Intermittent fasting is an alternative to the usual diets. It can also become a way of life if you think of the countless benefits that calorie restriction brings to the body and mind.

The different intermittent fasting types allow us to evaluate and choose the most suitable one for us, adapting it to our needs and lifestyle.

It is necessary to maintain a balanced and healthy diet, rich in vegetables and whole grains, and that provides all the macronutrients needed by the body, the right amount of fat (preferably vegetable) and avoid seasoned or salty junk food. All in all, however, you can eat anything, even taking a few whims from time to time.

Fasting has positive implications for the health of women over 50. Science has shown that reducing calorie intake prolongs life because it acts on the metabolic function of longevity genes, reduces senile diseases, cancer, cardiovascular diseases, and neurodegenerative ones such as Alzheimer's and Parkinson's disease. Also, especially for women over 50, it has multiple benefits on mood, fights depression, contributes to energy, libido, and concentration. And as if that weren't enough, it gives the skin a better look.

To start this type of "diet," you must first be in good health, and in any case, before starting, it is always better to consult your doctor. The female body is susceptible to calorie restriction because the hypothalamus, a gland in the brain responsible for hormone production, is stimulated. These hormones risk going haywire with a drastic reduction in calories or too long a fast. Therefore, the advice is to start gradually, perhaps introducing some vegetable snacks during fasting hours (fennel, lettuce, endive, radicchio).

As mentioned, in women, intermittent fasting works differently than in men. Sometimes it is more difficult for women to get results. Physiological and weight benefits are still possible but sometimes require a different approach. Also, intermittent fasting on non-consecutive days is better able to keep those annoying hormones under control. Various scientific evidence shows that to achieve fat loss, fasting must be tailored to the sex.

For women, in particular, there are specific biological truths about fasting that will prevent you from achieving your goals of a better body and fitness if you ignore them. But there may be variations that allow you to overcome these problems. Fasting can prove to be a convenient and effective way to optimize your health and make you feel better, but only if it is done in a certain way.

Fasting, after all, represents the easiest and, at the same time, powerful detoxification and regeneration therapy that we can offer to cells and the whole organism. Putting certain functions at physiological rest does not mean that organs and tissues go on stand-by. On the contrary, thanks to the absence of a continuous metabolic commitment, they can dedicate themselves to something else, activating all those processes of self-repair, catabolism, excretion, and cell turnover that only in the absence of nutrients can take place at the highest levels.

CHAPTER 3:

Who Can Practice?

After years of dieting, I discovered the practice of intermittent fasting.

I am a healthy and slightly overweight subject, but I have not taken lightly this practice, as old as the world. Don't do it either.

If you are considering starting an intermittent fasting course, please consult your doctor.

Together you can rule out any potentially harmful effects on your body.

As for me, I was tired of continuing to gain weight.

Gradually as the years passed, I found myself with a few extra pounds without having done anything special.

Simply my body was changing, but I didn't change my habits.

You can imagine the consequences on my active life and my appearance.

At first, I tried the Rina diet, Hara Hachi Bu, and the anti-gluten diet, but after the first results, I could not keep those habits up.

Also, the food restriction that has always characterized every diet forced me to make sacrifices that, in the long run, I have never been able to tolerate.

I do not say that diets are wrong, but since I discovered intermittent fasting, I have understood that the right solution for me was to stay fit and "lighten" the body from a decidedly disproportionate dietary intake in everyday life.

But why start this practice at 50? I'll explain it to you right away!

When we hear about fasting, our imagination leads us to a moment of deprivation, which we imagine involuntary, and which causes damage to our health, physical and mental.

Fasting makes us immediately think of hunger.

And hunger stimulates terrible memories in us that we want to forget.

But fasting does not mean having to go hungry.

Hunger and fasting, you will find out by experimenting, are not synonyms, nor do they travel together. Rather.

In my experience, the calorie-controlled diet reduces the food ingested and causes an annoying sense of hunger. Fasting is not.

The reason? Reducing the calorie intake for at least 14 hours reduces insulin and consequently the feeling of hunger and the desire for sugars and problematic foods.

Seeing is believing.

This is borne out by the previous study carried out by Jason Fung and published in his book "The complete guide to fasting," an exact text accessible to all, despite its rigor from a scientific point of view.

Fung can argue how food intake is directly related to the increase in insulin and, consequently, to the liver's storage, in the liver, in the form of glycogen, and in what we call rolls of fat, through fat cells.

So, it is possible to break this pattern by fasting, reducing insulin production and thus allowing our metabolism to burn fat, even those not immediately available.

What to take during the intermittent fasting period?

During the fasting period selected among the most common ones that we will see later; solid or sugary foods are not consumed.

Therefore, ban alcohol, carbonated drinks, proteins, carbohydrates, and fats of all kinds.

During fasting, we can ingest herbal teas, coffee, and water at will.

But without sugar or even fewer sweeteners.

During the longer fasting period, it is possible to take meat or bone broth, vegetables, together with vitamin supplements if you feel the need.

In my experience, during the fasting period, the only thing I need is to drink water.

The abstinence from fats and refined foods develops an authentic resistance that makes me overcome the days or periods of fasting without any difficulty.

CHAPTER 4:

Benefits of Intermittent Fasting

What makes it harder to get in shape after age 50? We encountered digestion problems, weak joints, and insomnia; the hazard for creating numerous illnesses increases. Simultaneously, losing fat, hazardous paunch fat, can significantly lessen your risk for such genuine medical problems as diabetes, coronary failures, and malignant growth. The discontinuous fasting diet for ladies more than 50 could fill in as a virtual wellspring of youth regarding weight reduction and limiting the opportunity to grow regularly age-related diseases. The life duration enhances steadily as calorie consumption is reduced (until starvation) and the diet period. Curiously, intermittent fasting can also improve life duration, even when small or no general calorie consumption reduction. In particular, intermittent fasting is a meal plan with a decrease in meal amount like every-other-day fasting. Similar to Calorie Reduction, Intermittent Fasting can prevent risk elements for diabetes and cardiovascular disease in rodents. Disorders accountable for mortality in rodents like cancers, diabetes, and kidney disorders are also suspended or banned by Calorie Reduction and Intermittent Fasting. A rising amount of physiological influence of CL (Caloric Limitation) and IF that can influence their capabilities to enhance health duration was discovered on rodents, monkeys, and humans. Noticeable factors between these are the following:

- Enhanced insulin tolerance that ended in decreased plasma glucose and better glucose acceptance

- Decreased amount of oxidative damage as designated by reduced oxidative damage to proteins, lipids, and DNA

- Enhanced confrontation to many types of stress involving heat, oxidative and metabolic stresses

- It enhanced the immune function.

The two principal theories for the aging influence of dietary limitation are the oxidative stress assumption and the stress resistance assumption. Because CL and some IF schedules include a decrease in vitality consumption, rarer free radicals are created in the cells' mitochondria and, therefore, fewer oxidative hurt to the cells. When retained on a CL or an IF diet, individuals extending from yeast and worms to rats and mice display enhanced resistance to various altered forms of stressors. This influence with tension is related to cells' improved strength in numerous reconstructed tissues to injury brought by oxidative, genotoxic, and metabolic offenses. The maintenance of stress resistance replies to CL and IF around a variety of species delivers robust verification that this procedure donates to the life duration- delaying the action of dietary limitation.

Effect on Cardiovascular System

According to the World Health Organization information, 17.9 million people die every year because of cardiovascular disorders, about one-third of all deaths. The utmost often disturbs individuals over 45 years of age. The death rate varies in both genders in any assumed duration of life. Among the ages of 45–59, men dominate, while after the age of 60, the death rate is more in women. These dissimilarities are associated with the cardio defensive influence of estrogens in premenopausal women. Variable and invariable elements take part in the progress of cardiovascular disorders. Age phases, sex, or hereditary components are out of our capability to control.

Moreover, smoking addiction, overweight, deficiency of physical activity, illnesses of lipid digestion, hypertension, diabetes, and unhealthy diet are modifiable habits. The presence of at least two dangerous bad habits improves the probability of the disease occurring. Therapy of cardiovascular diseases contains the modification of lifestyle, considering pharmacotherapy and invasive treatment.

The control of bad habits allows a decrease in death and pathogenicity, specifically in patients with unverified cardiovascular disease. With a healthy lifestyle, a balance exists, i.e., smoking cessation, enhancing physical activity, or guaranteeing appropriate body weight, all to decrease the danger of cardiovascular disease. Against the increasing diffusion of obesity in the world, diet modification is a significant changeable factor. Meals should be changed and aligned with a healthy Mediterranean diet. For instance, a good meal plan consists of a high presence of vegetables, fruit, fish, and only whole-grain bread. On the contrary, healthy habits are not allowed to eat animal protein, excessively salty foods (recommended daily salt intake less than 5 g), and to drink sweetened beverages. Also, it avoids the consumption of large amounts of alcohol. The consumption of spirits is a maximum of 10 g/day in ladies and 20 g/day in men. For various people, intermittent fasting is low restrictive concerning the conventional caloric limitation diet. It includes taking a typical, daily caloric consumption with short, stringent calorie limitation. It is possible to consume meals within this diet only in a determined range of time, day, or week. There are two ways to follow the IF diet that is time-limited feeding and alternate-day fasting. The famous three types of IF are

- 16/8 method

- Eat-Stop-Eat

- The 5:2 diet

The first one, also called the Leangains protocol, considers skipping breakfast and eating only for eight hours. Then this method includes 16 hours of fast and 8 hours when it is possible to eat. In a more severe methodology, the nutritional gap reduces to 4 hours. The 16:8 method is more popular and relatively easy to follow. The second one comprises 24 hours of fasting duration. Then one time, or two, a week, the meals are skipped for an entire day. The 5:2 method consists of consuming fewer calories, 500-600 calories, for two non-consecutive days but regularly eating for the other five days. Various studies of Intermittent fasting in both animals and humans verify the benefits in health and weight control. Moreover, IF decreases body weight and enhance cardio defense.

The cardio defense enhancement due to the alternate-day fasting diet is possibly linked with a limitation of fat tissue (in particular visceral fatty tissue), in-creased adiponectin amount, and decreased leptin low-density lipoprotein (LDL) concentration. In other studies, people following alternate-day fasting, after a period of dietary limitation, perceived enhancement in hunger within the day and enhanced satiety after a meal, which ended in consumption problems. Time-restricted feeding consists of consumption within a specific gap of time. The protocol may alter according to individual choices and lifestyles and include the restriction of fasting for too many hours (6-12 hours). This protocol may aid athletes in gaining the anticipated body mass for a specific sports grouping. Moro et al. submitted a trial on 34 resistance-trained males to a time-restricted feeding compared to a control group. After eight weeks of this treatment, the IF testing group encountered a significant decrease in fat mass. The fat-free mass remains constant in both groups (control and tested group).

The researchers observed a reduction in the arm and thigh muscle cross-sectional. Leg press maximal strength increased significantly. Also, the values of blood glucose and insulin decreased significantly only in the tested group. No significant changes were detectable for lipids (total cholesterol, HDL, and LDL), except for a TG decrease in the analyzed group. Time-restricted feeding is usually functioned daily and does not require suggested restrictions. The fasting gap may be at nighttime. In that way, it can assist some people in preventing night eating and follow a circadian rhythm.

Calorie restriction makes better flow-mediated vasodilatation in obese hu- men, which linked with a visible enhancement in insulin compassion, proposing a function for improved glucose metabolism in the beneficial influence of caloric limitation on the endothelial role. Mutually, the accessible data suggest that calorie limitation and Intermittent Fasting diets raise synaptic plasticity, grow the persistence of neurons, and enhance the number of neurons generated from stem cells. So, the dietary restraint makes better cardiovascular and cerebrovascular disorders in danger factors.

Caloric restriction and intermittent fasting have a positive effect on preventing various prevalent risk factors for cardiovascular disease and stroke. Individuals with insulin resistance (diminished glucose control) are generally linked with elevated levels of plasma glucose and insulin, then are at raised danger of cardiovascular disorders and stroke. Testing CL or IF on Rodents and monkeys shows increased insulin sensitivity, which would be predictable to reduce their hazard of diabetes and cardiovascular disease. Cardiovascular disease and stroke depend on high levels of low-density lipoprotein (LDL) and low levels of high-density lipoprotein (HDL). Reports on rodents, monkeys, and humans propose that CL can reduce LDL while increases HDL cholesterol levels. CL also reduces the levels of oxidative damage in the cardiovascular system, as described by diminished oxidative modifications of proteins and DNA and lower lipid peroxidation levels in the heart. Moreover, the limitation of calories decreases inflammatory procedure that probably causes atherosclerosis, as explained by lower levels of leukocytes and circulating tumor necrosis element levels.

CL can reduce, by repressing atherosclerosis, the hazard of cardiovascular illness and stroke. IF also recovers cardiovascular stress adaptation. For instance, when exposed rats on an IF diet to immobilization, the amounts of stress produced increases in BP and HR were less than those in rats on a control ad libitum diet. BP and HR each resumed to basal levels more quickly following the closure of stress in rats on the IF diet. Rats on the IF diet revealed initiation of the stress-receptive neuroendocrine system with the accumulation of stress. However, rats on the IF diet adjusted faster to replicated bouts of anxiety, as explained by decreased corticosterone replies analyzed with those on the control diet. As described, the heart rate alteration is enhanced in rats supported on IF and CL diets. Another physiological alteration is expected to decrease the danger of cardiovascular mortality.

Good Health Enhancement

All throughout history, various societies had discovered the advantageous effects on health and general welfare of reducing food consumption for definite periods, either for religious motives or when food was rare. The first extensive systematic study, published by Mc Cay et al. in 1935, highlighted the restricted eating diets and their capability to expand life-span. Mc Cay explained that feeding rats with a diet comprising of edible cellulose dramatically expand both the mean and maximum life-span in these animals.

Many studies have verified this consequence and extended it to mice and other species like fruit flies, nematodes, water fleas, spiders, and fish. So dietary changes affect life-span and health-span, then the time of our lives. We have a disorder/pathology-free disposition.

We will likewise analyze through which molecular mechanisms the points of interest, all in all, living beings, of dietary utilization changes are determined. Modification of this main dietary routine, now known as a caloric limitation, is the most effective way of expanding the life-span of mammals without genetically changing them. In particular, intermittent fasting has also been explained to extend life-span and have beneficial health effects.

CHAPTER 5:

Side Effects of Intermittent Fasting

Intermittent fasting is a significant lifestyle change, and hence when you adopt it, your body may react adversely. This adverse reaction is usually temporary and just a sign that the body adjusts to the new changes. You can also call these adverse reactions as side effects. The good thing is that most side effects that arise at the beginning of intermittent fasting are temporary and subside soon.

However, it is always better to know these side effects. There are some ways to manage these side effects better so that practicing intermittent fasting can become more comfortable.

Some Common Side-Effects are:

Cravings

It is widespread for you to have cravings. Either you go on a high-fat, low-carb diet or simply follow intermittent fasting, you will experience cravings in the beginning. These cravings are a result of energy demand created by the cells.

When you are living on a high-carb diet, your body keeps getting glucose at short intervals. The cells absorb the glucose only for their immediate use and would look for energy very soon. When your diet comprises refined carbs and sweets, your body gets an instant boost of energy.

However, this energy doesn't last long as insulin needs to stabilize the blood sugar levels, and hence whatever is not absorbed by the cells is stored as fat. Therefore, when the cells again need energy, your body doesn't have any, and thus you feel intense cravings.

When your diet comprises of fat, protein, and complex carbs, they release energy at a languid and steady pace. This means that there is neither any sudden energy boost nor energy is absent. Your cells keep getting power at a steady pace, and hence there are no cravings.

Your body will have to adapt to this change, and it can take some time. The best way to manage cravings is to eliminate refined flours, sweets, and empty calories from your diet. When you have a more regular diet, your body gets used to it and stops having cravings.

Headaches, Nausea, Lightheadedness

These problems are also connected with the issue explained above. When you adopt a fat-rich diet and follow long fasting periods, your body starts experiencing sugar withdrawal symptoms. Till now, it had been used for frequent insulin spikes and glucose boosts. These instances provided energy to the body whenever it needed. However, it also leads to problems like insulin resistance.

Intermittent fasting and a fat-rich diet put an end to this cycle. Your body stops getting a glucose boost at very short intervals, and that's why you may experience headaches, nausea, and lightheadedness. However, these problems are temporary, and these signs would go away in a few days as your body adjusts.

If you want to relieve the headaches and nausea, you can have unsweetened black tea or coffee. Green tea and unsweetened fresh lime water can also help you.

Heartburns and Flatulence

The changes in your eating schedule cause these problems. As we have discussed, the ghrelin or hunger hormone release is timed in our body, and it also leads to the secretion of gastric juices. These gastric juices can cause acid reflux issues that lead to heartburn. However, this problem will subside very soon as your body gets adjusted to your new eating schedule.

Here, the critical thing would be to stick to the new schedule as a failure to do so can again result in heartburns.

Excessive Urination

You may find yourself in a position where you may need to make frequent trips to the washroom. This happens when your body is dumping the excess water initially.

This is a common thing, and there is nothing to worry about. It would happen in most weight loss measures as your body tries to balance the new energy routine.

However, it is essential to note that your body doesn't just lose water, but it also loses minerals. It would help if you replenished those minerals to stay at the top of your health.

The easiest way to do so is to mix a pinch of rock salt in water and drink it when you come back from the washroom. You will have to be careful here. If you have high blood pressure or any other issue related to your kidneys, this will not be an advisable thing to do. Drinking electrolytes is safer and better in that case.

You must keep in mind that dehydration can be a problem initially, as you may rapidly lose water. This is a way for the body to get rid of the toxins. However, dehydration can cause many health problems for you, and hence that should be avoided.

But you must also keep in mind that you should not drink an excess of water as overhydration can also create problems.

A simple rule to follow is to drink plenty of fluids whenever you feel thirsty.

Intermittent fasting is a simple and effective way to stay healthy and fit. It is not just a weight-loss method but a way to achieve holistic health. These simple tips will help you get over the small obstacles that may get in the way.

CHAPTER 6:

How Intermittent Fasting Works

Before we can fully grasp how intermittent fasting works, we must know that there are only two states in which the body can exist.

Either the body is in the state of reserving food energy or utilizing or expending reserved energy. The primary goal of intermittent fasting is to ensure there is a balance in these two states.

Here is what happens during the fed state. When we consume food, the food goes through metabolism and then produces energy. Some of this energy is immediately spent, while some is reserved.

The reservation of energy is a vital responsibility of a hormone called insulin. So, during the fed state (that is, the eating period), insulin increases to break down carbohydrates first into simple sugar units known as glucose. This glucose is what the body immediately converts into its fuel, which is known as adenosine triphosphate (ATP) – this process is known as catabolism.

Secondly, in order to store more energy, it then builds up glucose in glycogen, which is a more complex form of sugar. This process is known as anabolism. This built-up energy is stored in the liver, and sometimes muscles get broken down later into glucose (the form of energy the body can easily use).

However, the body doesn't have an unlimited storage capacity to continue storing glycogen. So, what then happens when it hits its trench hold? The body initiates a process known as de-novo lipogenesis. This process is used to store more glucose by simply converting excess glucose into fat.

In this form, the body has an unlimited storage capacity. Some of this newly converted fat could be stored in the liver, but a bulk of the fat is moved and stored all over the body. This is known as body fat, and it results in weight gain.

On the other hand, during the fasted state (that is, the period without eating), the body carries out the opposite process. The body reduces the production of insulin, which we know is responsible for the storage of energy. Once the insulin level drops, the body immediately knows its state has changed, and as such, its process must change.

Knowing full well there is no food coming in and hence no external source of energy, the body is forced to visit its reserve. The body at this state begins to carry out catabolism. First, it starts breaking down glucose that was formerly stored in complex forms as glycogen.

The energy released in that process can sustain the body for up to 36 hours. If the body continues in this state, the body is further forced to start breaking down its fat reserve. This mode the body enters is called ketosis. It is the stage where the body switches from its usual and normal source of energy, which is glucose, to ketones and fat.

With this, the body can have the energy to function for days depending on the amount of already accumulated fat. This process would result in weight loss naturally.

When one intermittently fasts, they are only creating or maintaining the balance between the fed state and the fasted state. An imbalance may be in the side of always eating, which causes the body to have more calories than it really needs. Aside from that, it also continuously overworks the body as it continuously breaks down consumed food.

This could result in several health issues. So, in order to remain healthy, one must, from time to time, frequently allow the body to use up its reserved energy. This is absolutely normal as all animals do it to maintain their health.

How Intermittent Fasting Affects the Brain

The brain is a vital organ responsible for controlling every other part of the body. And it will interest you to know that the human brain makes up less than 2% of the total body mass. It is the principal seat of intelligence and is responsible for our personal and societal developments.

Among the numerous functions of the brain include; maintaining consciousness, memory recall, process data including languages, skill learning, and so on. So, the importance of ensuring that the necessary nutrients needed by the brain are provided cannot be overemphasized.

To keep the brain healthy and functioning at an optimal level, the brain uses up to about 20% of the calories generated each day. For such a small organ as the brain, one would think this amount of energy is too much. But the brain is always working, sending signals throughout the body.

The signals sent by the brain either bring about voluntary actions or involuntary actions. Even when we are asleep, the brain still works, although not as much as when we are wide awake.

If the brain needs this much energy to function, the next thing that might come to mind is that fasting would have a negative effect on it. But this is not true, as we will begin to examine how fasting works when it has to do with the brain. First of all, fasting plays a great role in the development of new brain cells.

When we intermittently fast, the brain-derived neurotrophic factor (BDNF) is triggered, facilitating the process of developing synapses and brain cells. Fasting also enhances serotonin, which is a chemical messenger in the brain. BDNF is commonly known to prevent stroke and depression.

Fasting increases these functions and a lot more of BDNF up to about 55 to 350%. Another way fasting affects the brain is it works to prevent neurodegeneration. We already know that fasting initiates autophagy, and during this process, beta-amyloid plaques are evacuated from the body, thus reducing oxidative stress, which might be on the neuronal tissue. Fasting has been reported to be one of the treatments for epileptic patients.

Intermittent fasting not only prevents degeneration but also enhances neuroregeneration and protection. This it does by boosting growth hormones, which act to prevent muscle depreciation. Lastly, fasting helps to facilitate mitochondrial biogenesis, which is known as the powerhouse of the cell.

The brain contains numerous cells and, as such, contains numerous mitochondria. A boost in mitochondria results in an increase of available energy in the brain. However, this will be discussed in detail below. Still, there is a wide range of beliefs that fasting causes starvation, leading to hypoglycemia.

This is the survival state of the body – instead of the body starting to convert saved glucose and subsequently stored fat in the body, the body continues to store up this energy and enters into a hibernation mode. At this stage, the blood sugar drops, and the body starts to shut down some of its functions.

The individual starts experiencing fatigue, shivers, low brain function in the form of forgetfulness, and lastly, fainting. While this might be true for extended unmonitored fasting, this is not the case for intermittent fasting. The reason is that one still eventually eats after avoiding food for some time. So, the body knows it has not gotten to starvation.

How Intermittent Fasting Affects the Mitochondria

Like we noted earlier, mitochondria are the powerhouse of the cells. Their health is very important to not only the cell but to the entire organism. To ensure the mitochondria (and the entire cell) remain in good health, dysfunctional cellular components eventually must be eliminated.

Also, the cell needs to perpetually be in homeostasis, and free radicals, either chemicals or organelles, cannot be allowed to remain in the cell. All these processes can be triggered by time-controlled fasting.

Intermittent fasting can also engineer the development of new mitochondria through the process of mitochondria biogenesis. This process is a result of some metabolic regulators, which include AMPK and PGC-1.

The regulators are responsible for not only building new mitochondria but also regulating mitophagy (the process where the mitochondria self-heals). They initiate the building of new mitochondria by sending signals to the body to increase the production of more energy in a stressful and energy-depleting environment (intermittent fasting).

To follow this command, the cell then develops new mitochondria (power plants) to produce more energy. This process has the effect of keeping one always energized and youthful.

Intermittent fasting also boosts mitochondria density. This is the ability of the mitochondria to not just produce more energy while making use of fewer resources but to be very efficient in doing it. This development is a result of a boost in NAD+ levels, which is one function of intermittent fasting.

The NAD+ is an enzyme that plays a vital role for the mitochondria to be able to produce more energy. Its presence in the cell energizes the mitochondria in its early stages of life. It also restores and replenishes the mitochondria during old age. It does this by initiating mitophagy as well as DNA repair.

Another key function of the NAD+ is the activation of Sirtuins. Sirtuins are charged with the responsibility of protecting the cell from stress. Like we mentioned earlier, during intermittent fasting, the body begins to burn stored up body fat instead of its regular glucose.

The breaking down of glucose leaves behind free radicals and produces higher oxidative stress when compared to breaking down fatty acids. So, we can say that intermittent fasting slows down mitochondria's aging process because it leads to the release of fewer free radicals and oxidative stress in the cell.

How Intermittent Fasting Affects the Immune System

The immune system is essential in the body as its health ensures the whole body's continued health. When fasting, stem cells are turned on. These stem cells play vital roles in rejuvenating aging cells, which end up prolonging their youthfulness. An example of this stem cell is the Hematopoietic Stem Cell (HSC).

Fasting accomplishes this process by shutting down Cyclic Adenosine Monophosphate (cAMP) dependent Protein Kinase A (PKA). the cAMP is a molecule messenger, while PKA is a bunch of enzymes. Both are responsible for the regulation of fat, glycogen, and sugar metabolism.

Once PKA is shut down by turning on the cAMP signal, the body knows to start mobilizing its reserved energy. And the minute the body begins to burn body fat, stem cells are activated. But it takes time for this process to kickstart.

This is because the body needs to finish burning all available glucose and all the glycogen it reserved before it can begin to burn body fat reserve. So, for this to happen, one has to engage in regular or long-term intermittent fasting.

Also, fasting could act as stressors that could be harmful to the body. But if it is done correctly in time, it can become a handy tool. Gradually exposing the body to stressors through intermittent fasting helps the body get used to and develop resilience against them.

So, the more one intermittently fasts, the more resilient to stressors one's immune system becomes.

CHAPTER 7:

Do's and don'ts of Intermittent Fasting for 50+ Women

The Dos

Dos of Intermittent Fasting requires that these steps be followed to make full use of it.

• Daily contact with your doctor is an essential part of intermittent fasting. Try always to follow your doctor's suggestions and avoid using your ideas, leading to harmful side effects.

• Plan your tight schedule. Those who do not plan will fail. Choose an appropriate time from your daily routine to work intermittently quickly. The best way to arrange an irregular schedule is to consult a physician.

• Ask your doctor to analyze your body weight and calorie intake so that you can suggest the proper fasting plan.

• Try to follow your doctor's diet plan during eating hours and avoid taking calorie-enriched food. You don't want to become a cactus! Stay Hydrated.

• Make sure you continue to drink water while limiting your calorie intake. Drinking water will cleanse your body and cleanse the blood vessels.

• If you cannot drink water in sufficient quantities, for some reason, try to take fruits and their juices which contain a large amount of water, such as orange and watermelon. Apart from water, tea, black coffee, and natural juice, these are good add-ons to keep you hydrated.

Monitor your Body's Responses

• Check your body's circumstances closely. Try to track your body weight on a weekly basis, and this will help you make a comparison and make decisions accordingly. Many people feel uncomfortable and tired when they first try intermediate fasting.

• Just make sure you don't lose weight by over-doing it. You probably know someone who started to do intermediate fasting and then became anorexic.

• Intermittently quickly to the degree that you could comfortably complete your daily work.

• Taking Vitamins Intermittent quickly will cause your body to have reduced vitamins. Taking the extra vitamins at the recommendation of the doctor to prevent this disease. Eat fruits that have large amounts of vitamins and minerals together with supplements. Avoid products that are artificially sweetened.

• Relax and enjoy the fun. It is hard for a person to spend time dreaming about all the donuts or hamburgers they will eat during a holiday. It can lead to irritation, stress, and depression sometimes. Avoid this by taking part in fun activities and talking to your friends. Try not to be alone and bored with a quickness. It ought to be a happy time.

The Don'ts

To optimize the intermittent fast effect, stay away from the things below.

•	Do not eat too much before fasting. According to experts, heavy meals before fasting is strongly discouraged. It can harm your health, especially your stomach, due to the slow-burning nutrition in fatty or oily food.

•	Always try taking the medium protein meal and low calories before fasting. At night you have natural sugar fruits, such as apple, mango, sweet melon, etc. Don't push too hard. Do not give your body priority over intermittent fasting if you feel ill or excessively exhausted at fasting.

•	Experts warn against fasting in conditions of health such as diabetes, cancer, and pregnancy. Precise steps must follow these conditions. Consultation with a doctor is essential for people with these health situations.

•	Don't be stressed out. Be calm and relaxed. Stress can increase your body's cholesterol level. Fasting is not necessary if excessive stress levels are induced in the body. Yoga and deep breathing are acceptable practices for stress relief.

- Don't do hard workouts. Lighter workouts such as yoga and jogging are always recommended to do during fasting. Remember that in the fasting state, your energy level is lower. Therefore, it goes without saying that you don't want to lift too much weight or run a marathon in this state. Be comfortable for a lighter workout.

CHAPTER 8:

What to Eat While Intermittent Fasting

We will look at some of the foods that you simply must include in your diet while you take up the fast.

Water

This is the most crucial element to consume when you take up the intermittent fast. Water can act as an elixir when it comes to losing weight. You must keep your body hydrated and ensure that all the toxins are dissolved and eliminated. All your organs need water to remain fresh and healthy; water helps keep these organs working smoothly. Drink at least 8 to 10 glasses of water a day and focus more on the fasting period. It will get a little monotonous, so the right idea is to consume fruit-infused water. This refers to water that has fruit and herbs infused into it. Fill up a jar with water and toss in fruit and herbs such as oranges, lemons, mint leaves, and a dash of cinnamon. Consume this every few hours. Remember that the intermittent fast can be quite taxing and lead to side effects such as headaches and nausea. In such a case, only water can help you out and put an end to these.

Fish

Fish can be considered a miracle food as it can significantly help with weight loss. According to dietary guidelines, people need to consume at least 6 to 8 ounces of fish every week. Fish contains a lot of nutrients. It is rich in fats and proteins. It is also rich in vitamin D., and this means you do not have to worry about denying your body these nutrients by taking on a fast. You do not have to reach for supplements if you can consume fish regularly. Fish is also rich in DHA, which helps in brain development. You will see that your mind is fresher and you can think well. Your productivity will increase, and stress will be curbed.

Avocado

You might wonder why avocado is on this list, considering it is one of the fattiest foods. However, you must understand that the fasting phase can take a toll on your body, and so you must consume foods that can keep you going. Avocado is rich in monounsaturated fat, which is excellent for those who tend to get hungry quite fast. It keeps you feeling full for longer. You will not find yourself reaching out to eat a snack. Avocado is quite versatile and can be added to your breakfast or lunch menu. Those who tend to include it in their breakfast menu are generally able to go without food for longer periods without complaining about hunger.

Leafy greens

If there is one type of vegetable that we remember being told to consume by our parents, then it has to be leafy green vegetables. As we know, leafy green vegetables are loaded with multiple nutrients that are great for your body. These include the likes of kale, broccoli, lettuce, etc. These are loaded with fiber. Fiber, as you know, keeps your body going when you suffer from digestive issues such as constipation.

You are sure to go through it when you adopt the intermittent fast. In such a case, it becomes that much more important to consume these vegetables to keep your stomach in good shape. Fiber also makes you feel fuller and not feel too hungry between meals.

Potatoes

As mentioned earlier, the goal is to consume foods that are filling and keep you going for hours, such as potatoes. Potatoes are rich in carbs that can keep you sated for hours. Make sure you either steam and mash them or roast them without the addition of any oil or fat. Deep frying them is never an option. Try to consume them with their skin on as the skin contains a lot of nutrition.

Probiotics

When it comes to digestion, both your liver and gut play a vital role. Both of them need a healthy dose of probiotics to function optimally. If you have an unhealthy gut, you might suffer from side effects such as constipation and even leaky gut syndrome. The best way to combat these is by consuming as many probiotics as possible. Some natural foods rich in probiotics include kombucha and kefir. Add these to your meals, and you are sure to experience positive benefits. An alternative is to go for probiotic supplements. Make sure you know which ones to go for. It would be best to consult a physician first.

Assorted berries

There is nothing better than consuming fresh berries in the mornings. They are loaded with antioxidants and vital nutrients required to keep your body healthy. Strawberries, raspberries, blueberries, and gooseberries are all great for you. Just toss them into the blender with some milk or yogurt to make a smoothie. According to studies, those who consumed berries regularly could remain within their ideal body weight and did not gain too much weight over more extended periods.

Eggs

An essential aspect of losing weight is building lean muscles. Lean muscles replace regular ones and prevent fat from getting stored. The best way to produce skeletal muscle is by consuming foods rich in proteins. A critical source of protein is eggs. Those who consume eggs for breakfast are better positioned to develop lean muscles and not go hungry before the next meal. Eggs can be quite versatile and cooked in any way you like. Hard-boil them the previous day so that you have a ready meal the following day. Simply toss them in a pan to scramble them. It only takes a few minutes to cook them.

Whole grains

One aspect of maintaining a clean and healthy diet is going for whole grains. The intermittent fast promotes these, as they are more comfortable for the body to digest and keep the system clean. They are also loaded with proteins and fiber. Do not limit yourself to the usual such as wheat and oats, and go for something different such as Bulgar, amaranth, and flax.

Legumes

If you wish to remain full for longer and not feel hungry or peckish too often, there is nothing better than legumes and beans. These cannot only be quite flavorful but also loaded with fiber.

The body does not easily digest fiber. The body cannot digest it but makes an extra effort to digest it, thereby drawing into the fat reserves. It is, therefore, best to load up on fiber to lose weight quickly. There are many options to pick from, including peas, lentils, green beans, fava, black-eyed peas, etc. These easily fit into soups and salads.

Nuts

Nuts are fatty, no doubt, but they contain good fat. Not all fat is bad fat as there can be some good fat as well. Polyunsaturated fats are said to be good for the body and can keep you feeling full for longer. You will not feel hungry if you munch on some walnuts or almonds. But make sure you make them a part of your meal and do not snack on them. Snacking on them can leave you feeling full and disrupt your meal plan. Do not worry about the calorie aspect. Nuts are not as calorific as you may have thought. They contain far fewer calories than some of the other fatty foods that people tend to snack on.

These happen to be superfoods that you must include in your diet while you take up intermittent fasting.

Foods to Avoid While Intermittent Fasting

Processed foods

Processed foods include biscuits, wafers, chips, cakes, and sugary drinks such as cola. These will only add to your woes and counteract your weight loss goals. Try to avoid these at all costs. Do not hit the aisles at the supermarket that carry these foods.

Junk foods

Make it a point to cut out all junk food from your diet. There should be no room for burgers, pizzas, and pasta that contain a lot of fat. It might be tempting to go for a cheat meal once in a while, but it is essential not to do so as it can lead to a habit.

Alcohol

Although wine is said to be relatively healthy, it would be best to limit it to just 1 serving per week. Try your best to avoid consuming hard liquor.

Although it is said that the intermittent fast does not tell you what not to eat, it is best to avoid these when you wish to lose weight.

With intermittent fasting, many people tend to follow their usual eating habits regarding the specific foods they put on their plate during each meal, expecting that they will lose weight just because they have fasted during the morning, night, and a part of the afternoon.

While intermittent fasting may improve metabolism and support digestive function that will ultimately enhance your ability to lose weight, the food you eat still counts. As you might have noted, the meal plans that I shared with you in this cookbook generally combine a range of healthy foods to ensure you get the nutrients you need without loading up on too many carbs. I did include a lot of delicious options that you can try out.

Just as there are a lot of foods that you can indeed include in your diet to help you lose that extra weight that is causing you concern, there are also some foods that you should always try to avoid if your goal is to lose weight.

Below, I would like to share some of the most essential foods that you should try to exclude from your diet to improve the results you can achieve when you implement the recipes and meal plans I have provided you within this book:

·   Fried foods, of course, should be at the top of my list. There is no doubt that fried foods are one principal reason for the world being so obese. Millions of people eat fried foods as much as every day. This does not only cause them to gain weight but also to experience a rise in cholesterol levels, be at a higher risk of heart disease, and more.

·   Fast foods, along with fried foods, since most chains that offer fast foods tend to deep fry their food in the worst types of oil and fat to make them tastier for the general public. Unfortunately, this also adds more fat to your belly, thighs, arms, and other areas of your body.

·   Corn is another food that isn't the best choice for people trying to lose weight. Sure, it is not an unhealthy food, but consider the fact that this is a type of grain that is relatively high in sugar. The sugar spike experienced when you eat corn leads to insulin release, triggering inflammation, and taking you one step closer to the dreadful complications of insulin resistance.

In addition to all of these, be sure to be wary of added sugars in everything you eat. For example, if you visit your local supermarket and grab a healthy bar to use as the food to break your fast, the fact that the word "health" appears on the bar does not necessarily mean it is truly healthy.

Always look at the ingredients of what you buy and what you will be putting into your body. Making your healthy energy bars at home might be a better solution as well.

CHAPTER 9:

Tips And Tricks To Know

Here are some tips and advice to get you started with Intermittent Fasting.

Stay hydrated. Drink plenty of beverages that are free of calories, such as water, herbal teas, during the day—avoiding a fascination with food. You must plan your fasting day around activities you enjoy, so you will not be thinking about food or obsessing over what you will eat next.

Resting & Relaxation. On fasting days, do not do strenuous exercises, while light physical activities such as yoga and walking around the house can be helpful.

Make each calorie count. Now that you have chosen a plan for intermittent fasting, it is necessary to eat every calorie as nutrient-rich as possible. Select foods that are rich in fiber, good lean protein, and healthy fats. Nuts, corn, lentils, poultry, pork, fish, and avocado are some examples.

Consuming high-volume products. You must eat nutrient-packed high-volume foods, but for snacking, also look for low-calorie foods such as melons, grapes, vegetables with high water content, fruits or popcorn.

Improve the flavor without the calories. Generously season your meals with flavor-packed garlic, vegetables, sauces, or spices and fresh herbs. These spices are low-calorie but rich in flavor and will help in feeling the hunger less. Select foods that are nutrient-dense during fasting time.

Consuming diets rich in fiber, vitamins, minerals, and other nutrients tend to maintain blood sugar levels stable and avoid nutritional deficiencies. A healthy diet can also lead to weight reduction and good well-being. If you want to the 16:8 intermittent fasting, here are the tips that people find useful:

•   Drinking herbal cinnamon tea throughout the fasting time because it can reduce the appetite

•   Consuming water periodically during the day

•   Watching minimal television to decrease sensitivity to food pictures that may stimulate a feeling of hunger

•   Working out only before or during the feeding window, since exercise will contribute to hunger

•   Try to eat thoughtful nutrition-packed food after breaking fast. Try meditation to encourage hunger pangs to pass throughout the fasting time.

Speak to your doctor if you're thinking about attempting intermittent fasting, particularly if you already have health problems such as heart conditions and diabetes. Expert advises trying to take it easy with the diet. The time window for feeding is shortened steadily over many months.

Also, as the specialist has advised, continue the medication routine. It doesn't interrupt the fast to take drugs and take the medication with calorie-free beverages like black coffee and water.

• What if you require food with medicines?

You may try to modify the fast in that case. It has been shown that overweight individuals can always do a lot of good even by taking medication with small portions of food. Simply work out a prescription with your practitioner that would support your wellbeing without losing the benefits.

You would like to ease into whether you are planning to attempt a fat fast or do intense intermittent fasting. If you are already consuming an unhealthy diet packed with quick snacks, fatty foods, and refined carbohydrates, you don't want to rush into these extreme fasts. One will find themselves in the bathroom for much of the day if you try to rush into fasting. Instead, by first performing a 16:8 fast on its own and keeping off the junk food, build your way up to doing these intense ways of intermittent fasting. Some literature speaks of doing a fat fast over a few days up to several weeks at a time.

• Your subconscious is the greatest barrier.

It's really easy to follow this plan. You simply should not eat until you wake up. Then you have lunch and dinner, and then you go on your day.

- Weight loss is simple.

If you consume less frequently, you will prefer to eat less in general. As a consequence, most people that pursue intermittent fasting wind up losing weight. You might be preparing large meals, but in reality, consuming them regularly is tough. Keep monitoring what healthy foods make you feel better during fasting, and keep cycling them. Intermittent fasting helps, but before a person incorporates carb cycling and calorie cycling, some people did not lose weight. By consuming a lot on the days, you exercise and eat less on the days you do not exercise, you cycle calories.

- Prepare to get a lot of water to drink.

For you, the safest lifestyle is the one that fits you.

4.1 Pay Attention to These Things When Starting Intermittent Fasting Over 50

One might find themselves grappling with hunger pangs as of a fasting novice. Don't worry; once the body gets used to intermittent fasting, these are going to vanish. Ensure that one drinks enough water, particularly throughout the fasting window, during the day. Water can help keep headaches at ease, which will encourage you to stay feeling full. Tea, black coffee, and low sodium bone broth are other drinks you can drink. Remember not to add milk or sugar to coffee and tea, or your fast won't do you any good.

Until you have achieved your fast, do not be pressured to overeat. Plan in advance: Load the plate with fresh, nutrient-packed foods full of high-quality lean proteins, fiber, and good fats instead of bingeing on anything in view. After the fast is over, these healthy meals will hold you sated and less inclined to overeat.

Here are some frequently thought-out questions for people over 50.

During the fast, can one drink liquids? Yes. It is good to have water, tea, black coffee, and other non-caloric drinks. Do not add the cream to coffee. There could be tiny quantities of milk or cream that are okay. They must be non-fattening. During a fast, coffee may be especially helpful, as it can curb hunger.

Is missing breakfast unhealthy? No. The concern is that there are unsafe lifestyles for most traditional breakfast skippers. If you make sure that for the remainder of the day, you consume nutritious food, so fasting is healthy.

When fasting, should one take supplements? Yes. Bear in mind, though, that certain supplements can function best when taken with meals, such as fat-soluble vitamins, so look out for that.

Can an individual exercise while fasting? Yes, easy workouts are okay. But remember not to overexert yourself. For women over 50, simple yoga, brisk walking around the house, and cleaning also count as a workout. Yeah, easy workouts are okay.

Would fasting trigger muscle loss? All forms of weight reduction can induce muscle loss, so lifting weights and maintaining your protein consumption is crucial. One research found that intermittent fasting induces less loss of muscle than a daily restriction of calories.

Can the metabolism slow down during fasting? No. Studies indicate that short-term fasting improves metabolism. Lengthier fasts of three or more days, therefore, can suppress and disrupt metabolism.

CHAPTER 10:

Fasting Mistakes to Avoid

You don't relax on it.

You are skipping breakfast. Skip lunch. And at 3 p.m. you are ready to eat your arm. "If you normally eat every 3-4 hours and then suddenly shorten, you're eating period to 8 hours, you're probably hungry all the time and discouraged," said Libby Mills, RD, dietitian at Villanova University's College of nursing.

"The decision to limit your meals may be motivated by weight loss. However, this is an opportunity to familiarize yourself with how your body really feels. We often eat every 3-4 hours and not always because we are hungry." You don't have to fast all week either. In fact, people on the 5: 2 diet eat regular amounts of healthy foods for 5 days and flip the switch on the other 2 days, reducing their calorie intake. A study of 107 overweight or obese women found that women who cut calories twice a week lost as much as women who consistently cut calories.

You consume too many calories.

According to Mills, you're not alone. "It can be easy to overeat when you break a fast, either because you're hungry or justifying yourself to make up for lost calories." She recommends using a scale of 0 to 10, where 0 means hunger and 10 is full. You need to be hungry before you eat, and you should stop eating when you're full, not just to clean your plate. He also recommends slowing down while eating so your brain has time to see when it gets full. "It can take 15 to 20 minutes after you start eating," says Mills.

You sabotage with soda.

Mills says the carbonation in soda can mask your hunger pangs, which can lead to you being overly hungry at your next meal and overeating. "Artificially sweetened drinks can also increase the satisfaction of sweet flavors, so if you eat a piece of fruit, it may not satisfy you.

He adds that these drinks can also contain caffeine, which can affect people differently. "A little caffeine can make you nervous and lead to sweet cravings. While other caffeine can mask your hunger pangs and delay it until the hunger is over."

It does not track your water consumption.

In general, you should drink 2 liters (i.e., 1/2 gallon) of water per day. "Water is part of our body's metabolic responses and is necessary for it to function properly. Hydration prevents us from confusing hunger with thirst," Mills notes.

When snacking, opt for non-starchy fruits and vegetables that contain water (yes, hydrating foods count towards your daily water goal!). Make sliced cucumbers, celery, watermelon, and oranges in the fridge or lunch box.

You are not eating the right foods when you break your fast.

Mills says eating enough lean protein (such as meat, poultry, fish, and vegetable proteins such as legumes), nuts, and seeds with each of your meals will help you feel full for longer. "Protein helps us feel full. Plus, when you lose a few pounds, protein helps keep your lean body mass metabolically active."

Another benefit, according to Mills, is that the fiber in fruits, vegetables, whole grains, and legumes slows down the digestion and absorption of the carbohydrates you eat, so you can stay full and energized longer between meals. "Even when you choose foods that contain protein and fiber, you get the vitamins, minerals, and nutrients you need while redistributing your calorie intake."

Your approach is too extreme.

Sure, you want to grab this diet trend by the lapels and run with it, but there's no need to starve yourself. Eating less than 800 calories per day will lead to more weight loss (with a significant increase in hunger) but more bone loss. That is not healthy, nor sustainable, in the long term. Not to mention, if you manage to keep your windows from eating too long, you won't be able to continue like this. Make smaller, more manageable changes, and always listen to your body.

You have caffeine withdrawal.

Who said ditch your morning Joe, afternoon espresso, or hot tea? None! In fact, coffee is not bad for you. Mills says that "a caffeinated drink, especially if it's hot, is a comforting bridge between meals." Remember, do not add sugar or milk if you drink your cup when you are fasting.

You are in your head.

Whether you stick with intermittent fasting for a week or a month, it should feel like a natural part of your routine. "Shifting your focus to be more intuitive about when you eat based on your feelings of hunger and satiety makes sense for a lifetime."

"Choosing foods that nourish your body with the nutrients it needs to stay energized shifts the mindset from counting calories to a focus on the quality of life." It is less a model of diet and more of a new way of thinking and consuming food.

Participate in intense and challenging training.

You can exercise, but not like the Hulk. It's hard to do your best in a workout if your tank is empty. Moderate exercise is important for health benefits, but if you want to exert yourself a little more, make sure you don't have hours to go before your next meal. Basically, don't go to the gym at 5 a.m. and don't break your fast until 2 p.m. Your body needs fuel to get through a tough workout and replenish its reserves after one.

You give up because you ate at the wrong time.

Don't throw in the towel, and don't beat yourself up. You don't undo all your work with one meal, but you can do it with a bad attitude. Take the time to reevaluate and make sure the schedule you have set continues to work with your lifestyle. Maybe it doesn't work for you anymore and now youwant to change your eating window or relax it a bit. It's okay. Also, you recovered by concentrating on your food choices and eating as many high-quality, nutritious foods as possible. If you have the right balance of protein, fiber, non-starchy vegetables, and H2O, you won't be hungry throughout the day.

Talk to everyone about intermittent fasting.

It is normal to want to talk about something new that you are excited to learn. However, understand that many people may not approve of intermittent fasting. They may try to discourage you and convince you not to try. Some misinformed friends may feel like it will ruin your hormones or put you in the way of eating a mess.

Never change things.

To find the best intermittent fasting method, you will probably need to experiment a bit. Once you experience the results you are looking for, it can still be helpful to make changes from time to time. For example, if, like me, you feel that the warrior's diet is optimal, you can still benefit from a 24-hour fast now and then. Or maybe a modified fast several times a year. It is often a good idea to change your method from time to time.

Eating too many carbohydrates.

A moderate amount of carbohydrates (between 50 and 200 grams per day) is optimal for most women. If you regularly eat more than 200 grams per day, it can be more difficult to fast. Sometimes on the weekend, I take a break from the intermittent fast. That one day, I can eat paleo pancakes for breakfast, put honey in my coffee, eat desserts, etc. I probably have more than 200 grams of carbohydrates, and it gets harder and harder to fast the next day. Keeping your carbohydrate intake low will make fasting easier.

If fasting is too hard, your hunger is affecting your behavior, and you feel like you can't continue, try testing your ketones to see if you're making ketones. Ketosis makes fasting possible. If you can't get into ketosis, you should eat fewer carbohydrates.

How to distinguish the hunger signals

I would like to emphasize that fasting is not just about turning off hunger signals. It's about learning to distinguish them. With practice, you will notice the difference between regular hunger, which is just a slightly uncomfortable feeling in your stomach, and hunger that you should honor, making you feel weak or hungry.

Some days I can go without food until 5 p.m. because I feel really good and the hunger doesn't bother me. Other days I decide to have an avocado or a whole salad for lunch because I don't feel so good and can't go on like this. Now I can do this with confidence because through practice, and I have been able to feel the difference.

Compare yourself with others.

It may take longer than expected to reach your goals. If you see someone else getting more obvious results than you, it doesn't mean that intermittent fasting won't work for you. It just means that your body reacts differently. Learn to focus on what you are accomplishing and don't let others' success put you off.

Eating junk food instead of nutrient-rich foods.

Whether you practice intermittent fasting or not, it is always important to choose your foods wisely. Consuming whole foods rich in nutrients promotes optimal health. I recommend that you make vegetables the majority of your diet. Add proteins, healthy fats, grains, and legumes if necessary.

CHAPTER 11:

Types of Intermittent Fasting

There are countless types of intermittent fasting.

There are so many reasons why follow an intermittent fasting lifestyle, and at least as many methods for doing it. Therefore, it is fundamental to set some basic definitions before we go deep in detail.

Fasting – giving up the intake of food or anything that has calories for a particular time frame. Usually, some non-caloric beverages and water are allowed.

Intermittent Fasting – to fast intermittently by adding fasts into your regular meal plan.

Extended Fasting – fasting for a drawn-out period. It will, in general, be cultivated for a significantly long time.

Time-Restricted Feeding – restricting your regular food usage inside a particular time window. This is meant to improve the circadian rhythm and general wellness.

Usually, people doing intermittent fasting are restricting their food time and increased fasting time. To have something like an actual fast, it would need to prop up for over 24 hours, since that is the spot most of the benefits start to kick in.

Now, first, let's have an overview of 13 of the main types of intermittent fasting, then we'll go deep into the 6 that better suit women after 50.

1. 24-Hour Fasting

It is the fundamental technique of intermittent fasting – you fast for around 24 hours, and a short time later have a meal. In spite of what the name may suggest, you won't actually go through an entire day without eating. Simply eat around the evening, fast all through the next day, and then eat again in the evening.

You can even have your food at the 23-hour check and eat it inside an hour. The idea is to make a very prominent caloric shortage for the day. Most of the benefits will be vain if you, regardless of fasting, binge and put on weight during the eating time frame.

Gradually and occasionally, you can decide to fast according to your physical condition and needs of the moment.

A fit person who works out constantly would require, to some degree, more eating time frames and few fasting periods.

An overweight person who is sedentary and needs to lose some more weight could follow an intermittent fasting plan as long as they can until they lose the overabundance of weight.

2. 16/8 Intermittent Fasting

16:8 intermittent fasting was defined by Martin Berkhan of Leangains. It is used for improving fat loss while not having to go through an extremely demanding process

You fast for 16 hours and eat your food inside 8. What number of meals you have inside that time length is irrelevant, yet it is recommended to keep them around 2-3?

In my opinion, this should be the base fasting length to concentrate on reliably by everybody. There is no physical need to eat any sooner than that, and the restriction has many benefits.

Many people think it is more straightforward to postpone breakfast by two or three hours and then eat the last meal around early evening. You should not get insane, and it is demanding to observe the fast. The idea is simply to reduce the proportion of time we spend in an eating state and fast for a large portion of the day.

3. The Warrior Diet

The Warrior Diet is proposed by Ori Hofmekler. He talks about the benefits of fasting on blood pressure through hormesis.

The warrior diet not only improves your body's physical condition and resistance but also grows your mental attitude and outlook.

The Warrior Diet talks about old warriors like Spartans and Romans who used to remain on an empty stomach all through the day and eat in the evening. During daylight, they used to stroll around with 40 pounds of armor, build fortresses, and bear the hot sun of the Mediterranean, while having just a quick bite. Around evening time, they would have a huge supper consisting of stews, meat, bread, and many other things.

In the Warrior Diet, you fast for around 20 hours, have a short high-power workout, and eat your food during a 4 hours window. Overall, it would merge either two minor meals with a break or one single huge supper.

4. One Meal a Day OMAD

The One Meal a Day Diet, also called OMAD, simply consists of eating just one big meal every day

With OMAD, you regularly fast around 21-23 hours and eat your food inside a 1-2-hour time slot. This is remarkable for dieting since you can feel full and satisfied once the eating time comes.

It is unmatched for losing fat; be that as it may, it is not ideal for muscle improvement because of time for protein production and anabolism.

5. 36-Hour Fasting

In the past, people would quite commonly go a couple of days without eating; they probably suffered and yet even thrived. Nowadays, the average person can neither stand to skip breakfast nor go to bed hungry.

For over 24 hours is the spot where all the magic begins; the more you stay in a fasted state and experience hardship, the more your body is forced to trigger its supply systems that start to draw on fat stores, bolster rejuvenating microorganisms, and reuse old wrecked cell material through the system of autophagy.

It takes, at any rate, an entire day to see major signs of autophagy. Yet, you can speed it up by eating low carb before starting the fast, rehearsing on an unfilled stomach, and drinking some homemade teas that facilitate the challenge.

For 36 hours is not that irksome, truly. You fundamentally eat the night before, don't eat anything during the day, go to sleep on an empty stomach, then wake up the next day, fast a few more hours, and begin eating again.

To make the fasting more straightforward, there are mineral water, plain coffee, green tea, and some homemade teas.

6. 48-Hour Fasting

In case you made it to the 36-hour mark, why not give it a try to fast for a straight 48 hours.

It is only irksome getting through the change of habits. Once you overcome this obstacle, which generally occurs around your usual dinnertime, it gets a lot more straightforward.

The moment your body goes into an increasingly significant ketosis phase and autophagy starts, you will overcome hunger, feel very mentally clear, and have greater mindfulness and focus.

The most problematic bit of any complete fast is around the 24-hour mark. If you can make it to fall asleep and wake up the next day, from that moment onward, you have set yourself prepared for fasting for a significant period of time with no issues. You essentially need to get over this hidden obstacle.

Going to bed hungry sounds disturbing; in any case, this is what a huge part of the world's population does daily. This could make you think about your own luck and feel thankful for having food anytime you want.

7. Expanded Fasting (3-7 Days)

48-hours fasting would give you a short ride in autophagy and some fat consumption. To genuinely get the deep health benefits of fasting, you would have to fast for three or more days.

It has been shown that 72-hours of fasting can reset the immune system in mice. However, studies on humans have not confirmed that conclusion. Also, there may be some issues in prolonged fasting that are not under severe medical control.

Three to five days is the perfect time frame for autophagy, after which you may begin to see unwanted losses in bulk and muscle. Fasting for seven or more days is not generally suggested. Most people do not need to fast any longer than that since it may make them lose muscle tissue.

Fit people may want to focus on three-four of these expanded fasts every year, to propel cell recovery and clean out the body. Notwithstanding a healthy eating routine without any junk food, I myself do it anyway four times a year because of their tremendous benefits.

In case you are overweight, or you experience the negative effects of some illness, then longer fasts can really help you get back in health. Fast for three to five days, have a little refreshment break and repeat the plan until needed. I'll never say that enough; if you decide to go through this kind of longer fasting, always be sure of what you are doing and consult a doctor if in doubt.

8. Alternate Day Fasting

Alternate Day Fasting, as for the 5:2 Diet, is a very common type of fasting. Are they fully considered as fasting, nevertheless, despite allowing the intake of 500/660 calories a day on fasting days? Well, yes, they are, since these limited amounts of calories are only intended to help extend perseverance.

To have a sporadic caloric intake will not enable the whole of the physiological benefits of fasting to fully manifest. It would limit a part of the effect. In any case, a strict limitation is important for both your physiology and mind.

Everybody can fast. It is just that someone cannot psychologically bear the weight of not eating. Fasting mimicking diets and alternate-day fasting in this respect.

9. Fasting Mimicking Diet (FMD)

The Fasting Mimicking Diet can be used every so often. Commonly, it is followed by people who cannot actually fast, like old people or some recovering patients.

Fasting mimicking diet has been shown to reduce blood pressure, lower insulin, and cover IGF-1, all of which have positive benefits on life length. Regardless, these effects are likely an immediate consequence of the huge caloric restriction.

During the Fasting Mimicking Diet, you would eat low protein, moderate carb, and moderate fat foods like mushroom soup, olives, kale wafers, and some nut bars. The idea is to give you something to eat while keeping the calories as low as reasonable. In most cases, again, this is more about satisfying people's psychological needs of eating than the physical ones.

Zero calories would be just as effective, and it would keep up more muscle tissue by increasingly significant ketosis.

To thwart the unwanted loss of lean mass, you can adapt the macronutrient taken in during Fasting Mimicking Diet and make them more ketogenic by cutting down the carbs and increasing the fats.

10. Protein Sparing Modified Fasting

Protein-Sparing Modified Fast (PSMF) is a low carb, low fat, high protein type of diet that helps to get increasingly fit quite fast while keeping muscle toned.

Lean mass is a significant matter of stress for healthy people, especially in case they are endeavoring to do intermittent fasting.

A catabolic stressor will, over the long term, lead to muscle loss; notwithstanding, the loss rate is a lot lower than people may imagine. To prevent that from happening, you have to stay in ketosis and lower the body's appetite for glucose.

PSMF is absolutely going to keep up more muscle than the fasting-mimicking diet, yet there's the danger of staying out of ketosis in case you are already eating many proteins preparing yourself for muscle catabolism.

11. Fat Fasting

The fasting Physiology and the ketogenic diet may be considered in a general sense equivalent, and both of them start the metabolic state of ketosis.

When you are dieting, i.e., in ketosis, you are using fat and ketones as a basic fuel source instead of glucose. This facilitates you going throughout fasting each day since you will be consuming your own body fat.

Some moderate types of autophagy can safeguard ketones and keep up their effects; nevertheless, it is not as amazing as macroautophagy, which requires restraint from all calories.

Fat fasting, you can have a pinch of black coffee, 1-2 tablespoons of MCT oil, or some margarine. Anyway, anything with carbs or protein in it like bone stock, coconut milk, coconut water, or the like will break the fast.

CHAPTER 12:

Myths About Intermittent Fasting

There are so many myths about intermittent fasting circulating in health books and on the Internet. These erroneous statements have created a stigma around intermittent fasting that causes people to avoid following this breakthrough diet. Learn to see through these myths, which are not true.

Fasting is Dangerous

This first myth is simply ridiculous. Everyone intermittently fasts as they sleep. Doing it at other times or for a few days on end is no more dangerous than simply fasting while you sleep. The body needs a period to perform autophagy, and it cannot do that if it is too busy processing food all of the time. Intermittent fasting gives your body a well-deserved break while helping you preserve your health.

Remember, fasting is not starvation. You can still eat. Don't confuse fasting, which is healthful, with starvation, which is dangerous.

Fasting Can Lower Your Blood Sugar Dangerously

The body can maintain its own blood glucose levels by releasing glycogen or sugar stored in the liver. This fact means that you won't go low dangerously if you stop eating for a spell. Instead, it will balance out and cause your body to start burning fat. The fat will keep you nourished and prevent fainting from not eating.

If you feel faint or lightheaded, you may need to eat. Be sure to listen to your body. Decrease your fasting period if you keep having dizzy spells.

However, if you are diabetic or hypoglycemic, you may need some help to maintain blood sugars during fasting. Ask your doctor how you can do this maintenance. Some fruit juice will technically break your fast, but it is necessary if your blood glucose plummets down.

It Will Cause Hormonal Imbalance

If anything, IF will balance your hormones. Doing IF wrong will indeed cause leptin and ghrelin, the main hunger hormones, to go crazy and make people binge. Then they will feel guilty and restrict themselves more. The hormones will get even more imbalanced. This effect can suppress a woman's ovulation and even stop her period. However, a woman who implements IF correctly by keeping herself nourished in her eating windows will not experience this at all.

It Will Destroy Your Metabolism

Your metabolism will run on whatever energy source is easiest. Sugar from food is the easiest, so your body burns that first. With no sugar present, the body turns to burn its own fat cells. Either way, your metabolism works. You cannot destroy it.

Some say that if you fast, you will overeat and then have even more trouble losing weight. This problem is psychological, not physiological.

Often people hate restrictive diets so much that they do overeat when they stop dieting, causing them to gain the weight back. Then, they are resistant to new diet approaches and have trouble losing the regained weight. Affecting over 80% of people who have dieted, this problem is pretty common. But if you stick with IF and nourish yourself properly, you won't return to overeating, and you won't have this problem. IF doesn't ruin your metabolism to the point where you can't lose weight again if you do gain any back.

It Causes Stress

Technically, fasting is a period of stress. But as Dr. Fung points out, it is good stress that causes your cells to do their work more efficiently and handle the stress of illness more successfully. Therefore, fasting will not cause extra stress.

The first week or so can be stressful because the approach involves change. Relax a lot and do things you enjoy or find soothing. The stress will pass.

Fasting Can Lead to Overeating

If executed with care, you can avoid the urge to binge eat later. It is true that fasting will make you hungry because of your body's hunger signals. The key here is to keep yourself well-nourished when you do eat. Use bone broth to stave off cravings during fasting periods. Also, avoid going on long fasts when you first start. Don't allow the temptation of food around you or have lots of easy snacks in the house as you fast.

Fasting Causes the Body to go into Starvation Mode

Starvation mode is a myth that some people believe causes the body to hold onto weight when it perceives that it is not getting sufficient calories. Look at any person who has starved themselves, and you will see rapid, immediate weight loss and wasting. That picture of starvation proves that restricting calories to dangerous levels will not cause weight gain but rather weight loss. Plus, fasting is not a dangerous caloric restriction or starvation, so it will not cause any unhealthy "mode."

Fasting Causes the Body to Burn Muscle

Because fasting stimulates the production of HGH, it builds muscle rather than destroys it. It only promotes your body to eat fat, not muscle. People tend to start losing muscle mass if they consume too few calories, or essentially starve themselves. But they will not lose muscle if they stay nourished and hydrated and eat well between fasting periods.

You Can't Work Out While Fasting

You can absolutely work out while fasting. If you have eaten well during your eating window and have some extra body fat, exercise will only make your body burn more. Your body will get the nutrition it needs to fuel the workout from your fat stores and the last meal you ate. Be sure to stay hydrated for energy.

CHAPTER 13:

Fasting and Exercises

Exercising gets your blood pumping, releases endorphins after and during workouts, and may help you burn extra calories. The number of calories you burn will depend on the type of exercise, duration, and intensity. However, this is generally a small amount and is nowhere near the calories you burn from the basal metabolic rate. Instead, exercise helps in other ways. In the case of intermittent fasting, it can help regulate your energy levels and deplete available glycogen stores, forcing your body to burn fat if it isn't already. Remember those old-school workout videos with everyone talking about "feeling the burn?" Very rarely will exercise directly burn fat. Fat only gets burned after glycogen stores are gone (which takes a while). Most amateur athletes never get to that level of performance. We sometimes hear that burning x amounts of calories (3,500, for example) equals burning 1 pound of fat. More specifically, you are burning 3,500 calories, which results in losing 1 pound of fat, more or less.

Many people feel that exercising on an empty stomach is bad for you. One way this could be true is by causing a significant drop in blood sugar levels. Here, people with diabetes need to be extra careful. The best time for them to exercise would be just hours after starting a fast—when food energy is still running high in the body. An exercise of any kind will naturally bring blood sugar levels down. If someone can't regulate blood sugar levels efficiently (diabetes), they run the danger of having a severe episode of low blood sugar. Otherwise, the body can detect that blood sugar levels drop and make an adequate response to metabolize glycogen. People who find it difficult to exercise while fasting may elect to "cheat" by having a small meal before the workout. Protein shakes are notorious for this, as they tend to be high in both carbohydrates and proteins. Mixing whey protein with water may run anywhere between 120 and 400 calories, depending on how much powder is used. Mixing it with milk will increase the calorie content significantly. But normally, protein shakes aren't required to get through exercise.

If you are already acclimatized to the fat-burning stage of a low-carb diet, you will find it easier to get through regular exercise even when fasted. Trying to get a full workout in during the first week of Keto will prove difficult. Trying to exercise in the middle of a fast is also hard because you will suffer from the symptoms of low blood sugar. People with diabetes will need to take precautions against them. Since a diabetic should be monitoring blood sugar levels regularly, they should schedule a blood meter test shortly before deciding to exercise. If their blood sugar is too low, they simply shouldn't do the workout. At the very least, they should eat something to get these levels back to a range that is healthy for physical activity. Like with fasting, the workout should be terminated if you experience any symptoms of increased dizziness, lightheadedness, vomiting, or loss of consciousness.

The types of exercise you decide on undertaking will depend on your fitness goals. A good general recommendation for people who wish to be healthier is resistance training at least twice a week alongside the recommended 150 minutes a week of moderate to intense aerobic activity. These 150 minutes can further be increased to 300 minutes to receive even more benefits. These include lowering the risk of cardiovascular disease, reducing the risk of cancers, and a greater increase in weight-loss potential from physical activity alone. Whether a full 300 minutes of exercise is sustainable a week while fasting will depend on the fitness level of the person, as well as what their fasting routines look like—for example, somebody who is doing the "5:2" Method may simply decide not to exercise on their fasting days. Others who fast daily by skipping breakfast (and fasting overnight) may decide to get the workout done after the fasting period is over. Breaking the fast with a small meal and then doing the workout afterward is a good option. Exercise gets a little trickier on those longer (1–3 days or more) fasts. The considerations are still the same, and the risk of a low blood sugar episode increases.

Aerobic Exercise

Anything that gets you on your feet and moving around is considered aerobic. In specific, it deals with raising your heart rate for extended periods. It comes from the word that means "with oxygen," causing you to breathe faster than usual while giving your body enough oxygen to flow in the blood. Walking, jogging, jump rope, cycling, stair climbing, and countless sports all qualify for aerobic exercise. Current American physical activity guidelines recommend at least 150 minutes of this type of exercise a week. One of the easiest things you can do is walk. Walking is virtually free in most cases and can be a pleasant change of pace. You can take your dog or a buddy along with you to keep you company. These are also called endurance activities because you should maintain them for at least ten minutes at a time. This key here is to get your heart working faster and your breathing to be deeper. You should be working hard but still able to carry on a conversation. These activities will strengthen your heart and lungs, which are, after all, very important muscles in your body.

Balancing

Balancing activities are so important for older adults to reduce the risk of falls. Tai Chi and Yoga are both excellent activities for assisting with better balance. You can find DVDs, routines online, or classes taught by certified instructors. Remember to work with your body and your current level of ability, and don't try to do an advanced routine if you have never mastered a beginner routine. And keep in mind that flexibility activities also help with the effects of arthritis. While you will want to explore the different types of yoga before deciding on the best for you, here is a yoga pose that anyone can do at home and helps to wake the whole body in the morning.

Stretching

As we age, our muscles begin to lose their elasticity. This is part of why rolling out of bed in the morning gets more difficult as we get older.

Stretching activities will help you to improve and maintain your level of flexibility, which will help you to avoid injuries to your joints and muscles.

Anaerobic Exercise

The opposite of aerobic exercise is the anaerobic kind. This covers different forms of resistance training, including bodyweight exercises, strength conditioning, and weightlifting. Also covered here are high-intensity workouts like HIT and sprints training. Anaerobic exercise and resistance training, in general, are good for creating muscle and strengthening bones. The nervous system also benefits from the mind-body connection used with resistance training. Resistance is effectively teaching the muscles how to interface with signals from the brain. Both anaerobic and aerobic exercise should be used together to get maximum weight loss results.

CHAPTER 14:

Fasting for Weight Loss

How to Fast

Intermittent fasting (IF) was sweeping throughout the fitness sector with increasing ferocity within the last few decades. Together with its increasing popularity, an increasing number of folks are becoming vulnerable to another means of preparing their daily diet and handling their nourishment.

With that said, even should you choose to utilize IF, then it will have enormous benefits in regards to dieting, especially if you're attempting to lose fat; that is, once I find it useful as a dieting plan.

When done correctly, it might help you:

· Handle feelings of appetite by letting you eat larger meals when you do consume

· Boost diet adherence by providing you additional dietary versatility

Handling appetite and sticking to a diet are critical in regards to your overall achievement and capability to attain your objectives.

Intermittent fasting helps you do this; nevertheless, whilst some individuals can fast for extended periods with hardly any difficulty, others may find it a little more difficult, especially when first beginning.

To help you out, there are a choice of ideas which it's possible to utilize to get the absolute most out Fast and make your trip a bit easier.

These are items that haven't worked well for me but also friends and customers alike.

With no additional delay, let us jump in.

1. Start Your Fast After Dinner

Whether you are doing weekly or daily, among the best tips I could give you would be to begin your fast after supper.

Doing so means you'll invest a large chunk of your own Fasting interval asleep.

Especially when employing a daily fasting installation like 16:8 in the event that you start fasting following dinner then:

· Spend 1 -- 3 hours watching television or other day activities

· Spend 6 -- 9 hours

You have already fasted for anywhere from seven to 12 hours, creating a 16 hour a whole lot more manageable.

This implies:

· Boost dietary adherence

· Easier lifestyle

· More manageable desire

2. Eat More Satiating Foods

The food you eat may affect your ability to stick with a diet and follow your own fast, and this is really where IF will help you big time.

Picture your regular fat reduction diet

· Eggs or porridge in the daytime

· Followed by a dull dinner of unseasoned chicken breast, sweet potato, and veggies

· Protein and water/milkshake after your exercise

· You then finish the day with an equally uninspiring meal at the day

If you are fortunate, you can scrounge enough calories to have a couple of handfuls of nuts a couple of times a day.

If you are feeling unsatisfied and far from content using the idea, you are likely to need to get it done all over again, again and again, and again till you reach your target weight in case you do not stop before then is.

And of course, the appetite and cravings which come in addition to this kind of diet.

Now envision your fat reduction diet using intermittent fasting;

· You skip breakfast rather opting to consume coffee and water (or some other 0 calorie beverage you need -- see point #4)

· Lunchtime rolls around, and you still eat chicken breastfeeding, but that time, it's acquired a tasty BBQ seasoning and can be accompanied by sweet potatoes and a side of vegetables with a dressing table.

· Protein and water/milkshake after your exercise

· It is dinner time, and you are outside for a friend's pizza and birthday is about the menu

In your diet, this could cause one to freak-out or, more difficult, maybe not show up since you didn't wish to mess up your daily diet but using all the calories stored from not eating breakfast, you consume your talk and understand you are still inside your calories daily.

· On days where you are not outside in the day, you have sufficient calories to add 1 -- two little bites (omelet or something comparable)

Here is the distinction between IF and other nutritional supplement protocols, the liberty to incorporate the foods that you enjoy, and normally eat a more pleasing and consequently satiating diet.

Good satiating foods comprise:

· Potatoes

· Yogurt

· Eggs

· Bananas

· Oatmeal

· Soups

Or alternative foods which you can eat a good deal of without absorbing a ton of calories

· Fruits

· Vegetables

· Legumes

This is not an excuse to go mad (stage #2); however, rather, it is a chance to make a fat reduction diet you like and will stick to over your long term.

3. Stay Busy

Boredom is your enemy.

It is the silent killer which awakens into ruin your advancement little by little, gradually wearing you down and pulling you back up.

Consider it for a minute.

How often has been drained lead one to consume more than you need to do, need to even realize you're:

· You are doing something dull in the office as well as the bites let from the kitchen have been beckoning

· You are at home watching Netflix, it is fine but not attractive, and you end up mindlessly reaching for your snacks

· You are waiting for the flight from the airport and wind up surfing the shops or sitting at the restaurants...ingestion

But what is it all about being tired, which causes one to eat?

You can invite dopamine, a chemical in the brain, such as this.

Dopamine is why you feel great when you reach a goal and also is accountable for reward-motivated behavior.

Interestingly, it has been discovered that ingestion can stimulate the release of dopamine and also consequently, the great feelings it supplies.

Over that, it is 'crap' food, especially those high in fat, sugar, and sodium, which are great in making you feel good.

This behavior can be seen in the present study (1), which demonstrates that subjects who had been tired ate more calories compared to people who were not, with further study (Two, 3) revealing;

"That boredom increases food intake [in] both normal and obese [topics]. "

It is not surprising that you just eat more when bored; you are almost hardwired to chase this dopamine high.

4. Blunt Your Appetite

Without a doubt, hunger pangs will set-in from time to time after fasting.

When this occurs, the trick is to dull your appetite, and also, the very best means to do that is by using 0 calorie beverages, which help supply satiety and keep hunger at bay till it is time to break your fast.

So long as the beverage is 0, you're great to go. Illustrations include:

· Water

· Sparkling water

· Black java

· Black tea

· Green tea

· Diet beverages

Recipes

1. Healthy Breakfast Smoothie

Preparation Time: 5 Minutes

Cooking Time: 1 Minute

Servings: 1

Ingredients

- 1 ¼ cups coconut milk, or almond or regular dairy milk

- ½ cup kale or spinach, or both (¼ Cup each) if you prefer

- ½ avocado, sliced into smaller pieces

- ¾ cup cucumber, sliced into smaller pieces

- 1 cup of green grapes

- ¼ tsp. ginger, peeled and grated

- 1 scoop Plant-based protein powder - Honey to taste

Directions

1. Orderly mix all the above-listed ingredients in a small bowl.

2. Blend them until the mixture is smooth. Taste it and add as much honey as you desire

4. Pour into a glass and serve.

NUTRITION: Calories: 117, Fat: 15 grams, Protein: 20 grams, Carbs: 5 grams

2. Avocado Egg Bowls

Preparation Time: 10 minutes

Cooking Time: 40 minutes

Servings: 3

Ingredients

- 1 tsp. Coconut oil

- 2 organic, free-range eggs

- Salt and pepper- to sprinkle

- 1 large & ripe avocado

For Garnishing:

- Chopped walnuts, as many as you like

- Balsamic Pearls

- Fresh thyme

Directions

1. Slice your avocado in two, then take out the pit and remove enough of the inside so that there is enough space inside to accommodate an entire egg.

2. Cut off a little bit of the bottom of the avocado so that the avocado will sit upright as you place it on a stable surface.

3. Open your eggs and put each of the yolks in a separate bowl or container. Place the egg whites in the same small bowl. Sprinkle some pepper and salt into the whites, according to your personal taste, then mix them well.

4. Melt the coconut oil in a pan that has a lid that fits and put it on med-high.

5. Put in the avocado boats, with the meaty side down on the pan, the skin side up, and sauté them for approx. thirty-five seconds, or when they become darker in color.

6. Turn them over, then add to the spaces inside, almost filling the inside with the whites of the eggs.

7. Then, lower the temperature and cover the pan. Let them sit covered it for approx. 16 to 20 minutes until the whites are just about fully cooked.

8. Gently add one yolk onto each of the avocados and keep cooking them for 4 to 5 minutes, just until they get to the point of cook you want them at.

9. Move the avocados to a dish and add toppings to each of them using the walnuts, the balsamic pearls, or/and thyme.

NUTRITION: Calories 215, Fat 18 grams, Carbs 8 grams, Fiber 2.6 grams, Protein 9 grams

3. Blueberries Breakfast Bowl

Preparation Time: 35 minutes

Cooking Time: 0 minutes

Servings: 1

Ingredients

- 1 tsp. chia seeds

- 1 cup almond milk

- ¼ cup of fresh blueberries or fresh fruits

- 1 pack sweetener for taste

Directions

1. Mix the chia seeds with almond milk. Stir periodically.

2. Put in the fridge to cool and serve with fresh fruit. Enjoy!

NUTRITION: Calories: 202, Fat: 16.8 grams, Protein: 10.2 grams, Carbs: 9.8 grams, Fiber: 5.8 grams

4. Feta-Filled Tomato-Topped Oldie Omelet

Preparation Time: 5 minutes

Cooking Time: 6 minutes

Servings: 1

Ingredients

- 1 tbsp. coconut oil

- 2 pcs eggs

- 1½ tbsp. milk

- A dash of salt and pepper

- ¼ cup tomatoes, sliced into cubes

- 2 tbsps. feta cheese, crumbled

Directions

1. Beat the eggs with pepper, salt, milk, and the remaining spices.

2. Pour the mixture into a heated pan with coconut oil.

3. Stir in the tomatoes and cheese. Cook for 6 minutes or until the cheese melts.

NUTRITION: Calories: 335, Fat: 28.4 grams, Protein: 16.2 grams, Carbs: 4.5 grams, Fiber: 0.8 grams

5. Carrot Breakfast Salad

Cooking time: 4 hours

Preparation Time: 5 minutes

Servings: 4

Ingredients

- 2 tbsps. olive oil
- 2 lbs. baby carrots, peeled and halved
- 3 garlic cloves, minced
- 2 yellow onions, chopped
- ½ cup vegetable stock
- 1/3 cup tomatoes, crushed
- A pinch of salt and black pepper

Directions

1. In your slow cooker, combine all the ingredients, cover, and cook on high for 4 hours.

2. Divide into bowls and serve for breakfast.

NUTRITION: Calories: 437, Protein: 2.39 grams, Fat: 39.14 grams, Carbs: 23.28 grams

CHAPTER 15:

Fasting for Metabolism/Inflammation

How to Fast

Intermittent fasting has been shown to be a powerful tool in lowering chronic inflammation and improving health. We use it with all our patients at NUTRiBULLET, especially those over 50 who are more susceptible to chronic inflammation. Although it may seem odd that you can improve your health by not eating, fasting, experts say, is the simplest, most inexpensive way to take care of your body.

Read on to find out how many different ways intermittent fasting can help you feel better and live longer (and maybe lose a few pounds!).

Inflammation

The most efficient way to lower chronic inflammation is to fast intermittently for at least 12 hours every day. When we eat, our body uses glucose (sugar) from recently eaten foods as fuel. But if there are no more sugars in the bloodstream, the body can then turn to fat stores and use these as fuel. This process is called ketosis and helps the body burn fat, turning it into energy instead of storing it in dangerous areas of your body like your belly and liver.

As your body uses up the available fat stores, it starts breaking down other tissues in order to get the energy it needs to survive. This process involves the creation of what we call toxic byproducts that must be removed from your body, or they can cause damage. This is where antioxidants like Vitamins A, C, and E come in; they help clear out these toxic byproducts and keep your body healthy and young.

The same process that happens when you fast have a similar result as exercising- it burns calories! It's just that with fasting, you don't have to go for a run or lift weights; just don't eat for 12 hours over the course of a day. It's pretty simple, really.

Inflammation is a broad term that describes a wide variety of health problems ranging from mild to severe. These range from allergies, asthma, and eczema to rheumatoid arthritis, irritable bowel syndrome, and autoimmune issues. There are many more, but we won't go into them here- just trust us when we say that fasting will help you feel better in more ways than you can probably imagine!

Recipes

6. Zuppa Toscana with Cauliflower

Preparation time: 5 minutes

Cooking time: 25 minutes

Serving: 4

Ingredients:

- 1 lb. ground Italian sausage

- 6 cups homemade low-sodium chicken stock

- 2 cups cauliflower florets - 1 onion, finely chopped

- 1 cup kale, stemmed and roughly chopped

- 1 (14.5-ounce) can of full-fat coconut milk

- ¼ tsp. sea salt

- ¼ tsp. freshly cracked black pepper

Directions:

1.   On the Instant Pot, press "Sauté" and add the Italian ground sausage. Cook until brown, stirring occasionally and breaking up the meat with a wooden spoon.

2.   Add the remaining ingredients except for the kale and coconut milk and stir until well combined.

3.   Cover and cook for 10 minutes on high pressure. When done, release the pressure naturally and remove the lid. Stir in the kale and coconut milk. Cover and sit for 5 minutes or until the kale has wilted. Serve and enjoy!

Nutrition:

Calories 653 Carbohydrates 8g

Protein 26g Fat 4g

7. Pork Carnitas

Preparation time: 20 minutes

Cooking time: 1 hour

Serving: 4

Ingredients:

- 6 medium garlic cloves, minced
- 2 tsps. ground cumin - 1 tsp. smoked paprika
- 3 chipotle peppers in adobo sauce, minced
- 1 tsp. dried oregano - 2 bay leaves
- 1 cup homemade low-sodium chicken broth
- Fine sea salt and freshly cracked black pepper
- 2 tbsps. of olive oil
- 2 ½ lbs. boneless pork shoulder, cut into 4 large pieces

Directions:

1. Season the pork shoulder with sea salt, black pepper, ground cumin, dried oregano, and smoked paprika.

2. On the Instant Pot, press "Sauté" and add the olive oil.

3. Once hot, add the pork pieces and sear for 4 minutes per side or until brown.

4. Add the remaining ingredients inside your Instant Pot. Cover and cook for 80 minutes on high pressure. When done, quick release the pressure and remove the lid. Carefully shred the pork using two forks and continue to stir until well coated with the liquid. Remove the bay leave and adjust the seasoning if necessary. Serve and enjoy!

Nutritional Information:

Calories 170 Carbohydrates 2g Protein 4g Fat 8g

8. Garlic Butter Beef Steak

Preparation time: 5 minutes

Cooking time: 15 minutes

Serving: 2

Ingredients:

- 1 lb. beef sirloin steaks - ½ cup red wine

- 4 tbsps. unsalted butter

- 2 tbsps. fresh parsley, finely chopped

- 4 medium garlic cloves, peeled and minced

- Fine sea salt and freshly cracked black pepper

Directions:

1.   Season the beef steaks with sea salt and freshly cracked black pepper.

2.   On the Instant Pot, press "Sauté" and add the butter. Once melted, add the beef steaks and sear for 2 minutes per side or until brown. Pour in the red wine and fresh parsley. Cover and cook for 12 minutes on high pressure. When done, release the pressure naturally and carefully remove the lid. Top the steak with the butter sauce. Serve and enjoy!

Nutrition:

Calories 337 Carbohydrates 2.5g Protein 34.5g Fat 18.7g

9. Instant Pot Teriyaki Chicken

Preparation time: 5 minutes

Cooking time: 35 minutes

Serving: 4

Ingredients

- 1/2 cup soy sauce - 1/2 cup water
- 1/2 cup brown sugar - 2 tbsps. rice wine vinegar
- 1 tbsp. mirin (Japanese sweet wine)
- 1 tbsp. sake - 1 tbsp. minced garlic
- 1 dash freshly cracked black pepper
- 1 lb. skinless, boneless chicken

Directions

1. Combine soy sauce, brown sugar, water, rice wine vinegar, sake, mirin, pepper, and garlic in a bowl to prepare the sauce.

2. Put chicken in an electric pressure cooker (such as Instant Pot(R)). Pour the sauce over.

3. Close lid and lock. Set to Meat function, with the timer on to 12 minutes. Give 10-15 minutes for pressure to build.

4. Gently release pressure with the quick-release method according to manufacturer's instructions, for 5 minutes. Remove lid. Insert the instant-read thermometer into the middle of the chicken and make sure to reach at least 165°F (74°C). If not hot enough, cook for 2-4 more minutes. Take chicken out from the cooker. Shred or cut up. Mix with sauce from the pot.

Nutrition:

Calories 259 Carbohydrates 33.1g Protein 24.3g Fats 2.3g

10. Teriyaki Salmon

Preparation time: 15 minutes

Cooking time: 5 minutes

Serving: 2

Ingredients:

- 3 tbsps. lime juice - 2 tbsps. olive oil

- 2 tbsps. reduced-sodium teriyaki sauce

- 1 tbsp. balsamic vinegar

- 1 tbsp. Dijon mustard - 1 tsp. garlic powder

- 6 drops hot pepper sauce

- 6 uncooked jumbo salmon

Directions

1.   Mix together all ingredients except the salmon in a big zip-lock plastic bag, then put in the shrimp. Seal the zip lock bag and turn to coat the salmon. Keep in the fridge for an hour and occasionally turn.

2.   Drain the marinated salmon and discard marinade. Broil the salmon 4 inches from heat for 3 to 4 minutes per side or until the salmon turn pink in color.

Nutrition:

Calories 93 Carbohydrates 3g Protein 13g Fats 4g

CHAPTER 16:

Fasting for Body Detoxification

How to fast

Short-term fasting is used to detoxify the body and can be effective in improving the body's immune system. In contrast, a longer fast can be used to totally regenerate the entire system through autolysis and rejuvenation (self-digestion and self-regeneration).

Procedures:

1. A "water only" fast is defined as not eating or drinking anything except water for up to two days. Water has no calories or other nutrients that the body needs, so it is less likely to trigger withdrawal symptoms. After the fast, you can slowly add fruits and vegetables to a healthy diet plan.

2. A "juice only" fast is defined as not eating or drinking anything except fresh fruit and vegetable juices for up to a week. Some doctors recommend that you do not exceed 4-5 days on this type of fast, but there is no reason why you cannot go longer if your health care professional feels it is safe for you to do so. After the fast, gradually introduce solid foods in small amounts using a healthy diet plan.

3. A "juice plus water" fast is defined as not eating or drinking anything except fresh fruit and vegetable juices, plus one glass of water (8 oz) per day for up to a week. This type of fast allows you to detoxify and lose weight while getting needed nutrients from the foods that you are taking in. After the fast, gradually introduce solid foods in small amounts using a healthy diet plan.

4. A "juice plus water" extended fast is defined as not eating or drinking anything except fresh fruit and vegetable juices, plus one glass of water (8 oz) per day, for up to two weeks. This type of fast allows you to detoxify and lose weight while getting needed nutrients from the foods that you are taking in. After the fast, gradually introduce solid foods in small amounts using a healthy diet plan.

5. A "juice plus water" juice fast is defined as not eating or drinking anything except fresh fruit and vegetable juices, plus one glass of water (8 oz) per day, for up to one month. This type of fast can help your body regenerate itself through autolysis and rejuvenation (self-digestion and self-regeneration). An extended juice fast should only be undertaken under the supervision of a health care professional because it puts your body under great stress. I do not recommend extended juice fasts for most people.

6. A "water only" water fast is defined as not eating or drinking anything except water for more than two days and up to a month. Water fasting allows the body to detoxify itself while also losing weight and improving the immune system. This type of fast should only be undertaken under

the supervision of a health care professional because it puts your body under great stress. I do not recommend this type of fast for most people.

7. The total diet replacement program includes juices, protein shakes, soups, and supplements which are used during one or more days in combination with water fasting (no solid foods). This is not really a fast, but it can be an effective way to regain control over your body while losing weight and improving the immune system. This type of fast should only be undertaken under the supervision of a health care professional because it puts your body under great stress. I do not recommend this type of fast for most people.

Recipes

11. Beet Blast Smoothie

Preparation Time: 5 minutes

Cooking Time: 0 minutes

Servings: 1

Ingredients:

- 1½ cups unsweetened plant-based milk
- 1 Granny Smith apple, peeled, cored, and chopped
- 1 cup chopped frozen beets
- 1 cup frozen blueberries
- ½ cup frozen cherries
- ¼-inch fresh ginger root, peeled

Directions:

1. In a blender, combine all the ingredients and blend until smooth.

2. Serve immediately or store in the freezer in a resalable jar.

Nutrition:

- Calories: 324
- Total fat: 5g
- Carbohydrates: 70g
- Fiber: 15g
- Protein: 5g
- Calcium: 72%
- Vitamin D: 38% Vitamin B12: 0%
- Iron: 15% Zinc: 4%

12. Green Power Smoothie

Preparation Time: 5 minutes

Cooking Time: 0 minutes

Servings: 1

Ingredients:

- 3 cups fresh spinach

- 1½ cups frozen pineapple

- 1 cup unsweetened plant-based milk

- 1 cup fresh kale

- 1 Granny Smith apple, peeled, cored, and chopped

- ½ small avocado, pitted and peeled

- ½ tsp. spirulina - 1 tbsp. hemp seeds

Directions:

1. In a blender, combine all the ingredients and blend until smooth.

2. Serve immediately or store in the freezer in a resalable jar.

Nutrition: Calories: 431

- Total fat: 16g Carbohydrates: 70g Fiber: 17g Protein: 13g

- Calcium: 67% Vitamin D: 25% Vitamin B12: 31%

- Iron: 41% Zinc: 15%

13. Tropical Bliss Smoothie

Preparation Time: 5 minutes

Cooking Time: 0 minutes

Servings: 1

Ingredients:

- 2 cups frozen pineapple

- 1 banana

- 1¼ cups unsweetened coconut milk

- ¼ cup frozen coconut pieces

- ½ tsp. ground flaxseed

- 1 tsp. hemp seeds

Directions:

1. In a blender, combine all the ingredients and blend until smooth.

2. Serve immediately or store in the freezer in a resalable jar.

Nutrition:

- Calories: 396   Total fat: 14g Carbohydrates: 71g Fiber: 11g

- Protein: 6g Calcium: 64% Vitamin D: 31% Vitamin B12: 3%

- Iron: 19% Zinc: 7%

14. Very Berry Antioxidant Smoothie

Preparation Time: 5 minutes

Cooking Time: 0 minutes

Servings: 1

Ingredients:

- 1 banana

- 1¼ cups unsweetened plant-based milk

- ½ cup frozen strawberries

- ½ cup frozen blueberries

- ½ cup frozen raspberries

- 3 pitted Medjool dates

- 1 tbsp. hulled hemp seeds

- ½ tbsp. ground flaxseed

- 1 tsp. ground chia seeds

Directions:

1. In a blender, combine all the ingredients and blend until smooth.

2. Serve immediately or store in the freezer in a resalable jar.

Nutrition:

- Calories: 538 Total fat: 11g

- Carbohydrates: 111g

- Fiber: 21g Protein: 10g

- Calcium: 75%

- Vitamin D: 31%

- Vitamin B12: 8%

- Iron: 26%

- Zinc: 13%

15. Green Pineapple

Preparation time: 5 minutes

Cooking time: 0 minutes

Serving: 3

Ingredients:

- 1/2 of a pineapple
- 1 broccoli, diced
- 1 cup water
- 1 long cucumber, diced
- A dash of salt
- 1 kiwi, diced

Directions

1. Add kiwi, cucumber, pineapple, broccoli, and water in a blender.

2. Add the salt and blend until smooth.

3. Serve.

Nutrition:

Calories 251 Fats 0.4g

Proteins 0.5g Carbohydrates 22g

CHAPTER 17:

Fasting for Mental Health

How to fast

Don't eat anything for breakfast. Eat a light lunch of soup or other clear liquids. Eat your main meal between 1 p.m. and 3 p.m. Avoid snacking in the afternoon and evening. Go to bed soon after dinner, and don't eat before you go to sleep.

Why? Intermittent fasting is a way of eating that cycles between not eating, sometimes for 24 hours at a time, and then not eating again until the following day.

Since starting intermittent fasting, I have learned that the most effective way to do it is to eat a light lunch and then not eat again until breakfast the next day.

When you're not fasting, you can eat whatever you want, but you can't over-eat. That's because when you start eating again after fasting, your body releases a lot of insulin, which helps to turn any excess food into stored fat. So, if you're not fasting, try to keep your meals small and 'balanced.'

One of the best things about intermittent fasting is that it makes it easier for you to stick to a healthy, balanced diet. You'll find yourself naturally eating less processed foods, snacks, and sweets because they just aren't there for you to eat.

Fasting is also effective at reducing cravings for food and alcohol. It's helped me drink a lot less during the week.

When I'm not fasting on the weekends, I make sure that I only have three meals a day plus two 'mini-meals' in between.

For example, I have a coffee with almond milk and two squares of dark chocolate in the morning. Then I have a small piece of fruit around noon and an evening meal that's mostly vegetables.

I feel physically lighter when I don't eat much at night or in the afternoon.

Before you start any new diet or exercise program, it's always best to talk to your doctor first. In my case, my doctor is happy for me to try intermittent fasting because, as far as he's concerned, it is not really a diet but an eating pattern that can help me lose weight gradually (I started at 13st 7lb).

I'm also able to do intermittent fasting because I don't have any history of diabetes, high blood pressure, or heart disease in my family.

The only thing I've noticed since starting intermittent fasting is that sometimes, after the second day of not eating anything, I feel a bit tired and achy. But that feeling usually goes away after the morning of the third day.

Recipes

16. Blueberry-lemon Smoothie

Preparation time: 3 minutes;

Cooking time: 2 minutes;

Servings: 2

Ingredients:

- ½ banana – ½ - 1 cup frozen blueberries

- 1 cup lemon yogurt

- ¼ cup grape juice - 1 tsp. honey

Directions:

1.   Using a blender, add in all ingredients. Process until you obtain a smooth consistency.

2.   Pour into two glasses and serve as a quick breakfast.

Nutrition:

Calories: 261, Fat: 2.5g, Protein: 6g, Carbs: 57g

17. Strawberry-banana Smoothie

Preparation time: 3 minutes;

Cooking time: 2 minutes;

Servings: 2

Ingredients:

- 1 banana

- 1 cup frozen and sliced strawberries

- 1 cup frozen vanilla yogurt

- ¼ cup orange juice

- 1 tsp. honey

Directions:

1. Place all ingredients in a blender and blend until smooth.

2. Pour into two glasses and serve as a quick breakfast.

Nutrition:

Calories: 248, Fat: 4g, Protein: 4g, Carbs: 50g

18. Spinach with Baked Eggs

Preparation time: 5 minutes;

Cooking time: 15 minutes;

Servings: 2

Ingredients:

- 2 tsps. olive oil
- 10 cups spinach
- 2 tsps. garlic
- 1 cup cheese, shredded
- 2 eggs

Directions:

1. Preheat the oven to 325 F

2. In a skillet, heat oil, add 1 tsp. garlic, spinach and sauté for 3-4 minutes Add ¼ cup cheese and divide mixture into 2 ramekins

4. Crack one egg over each spinach mixture

5. Bake for 12-15 minutes Add salt, pepper and serve

Nutritional Info:

Calories: 205.7, Fat: 13.5g, Carbs: 3.6g, Protein: 17.5g

19. Quinoa Berry Bowl

Preparation time: 5 minutes;

Cooking time: 10 minutes;

Servings: 4

Ingredients:

- 1 cup cooked quinoa
- 1 tbsp. coconut oil
- 1 tbsp. coconut sugar
- ½ cup berries
- Coconut milk

Directions:

1. In a saucepan, cook quinoa

2. Drizzle coconut oil and add coconut sugar, mix well. Add berries and strawberries

4. Drizzle a little bit of coconut milk and serve

Nutrition:

Calories: 224.7, Fat: 2.5g, Carbs: 42.8g, Protein: 4.4g

20. Blueberry Muffins

Preparation time: 5 minutes;

Cooking time: 25 minutes;

Servings: 12

Ingredients:

- 2 eggs

- 1 cup applesauce

- ½ maple syrup

- ½ cup avocado oil

- ½ cup vanilla extract

- 1 tsp. cinnamon

- 1 tsp. baking powder

- ¼ tsp. baking soda

- 1 cup wheat flour, whole

- 1 cup blueberries

Directions:

1. Preheat the oven to 325 F

2. In a bowl, combine all ingredients together, whisk well

3. Add blueberries and scoop batter into 12 muffin cups

4. Bake for 20-25 minutes

5. When ready, remove and serve

Nutrition:

Calories: 217, Protein: 3g, Carbs: 33g, Fat: 8g

CHAPTER 18:

Fasting for Longevity

How to Fast

Longevity really means long life, and aside from genetics that you can't really control, there are only a few areas that you can modify to give yourself a long life: diet, lifestyle, and exercise. Fasting promotes a healthier lifestyle and encourages better habits. Since it is a natural way to lose weight, it will be something you can longer. You could try out a complicated diet involving meal replacements and supplements, but at the end of the day, this might result in you gaining weight faster than you lost it. The fluctuation of weight gain and loss isn't always good for our bodies. Even if you do manage to keep up with it, it may not be a good long-term solution. To live a long and healthy life, you have to make healthy choices. Train your body to burn fat and detoxify constantly, and you will be doing your very best to try and achieve longevity through fasting.

Recipes

21. Beef & Barley Soup

Preparation Time: 10 min.

Cooking Time: 50 min.

Servings: 8

Ingredients:

½ cup parsley, finely chopped

½ tsp. thyme, dried

1 cup wheat barley, hulled

1 lb. ground beef

1 large onion, diced

1 tbsp. extra virgin olive oil

1 tsp. salt

2 large stalks celery, diced

3 bay leaves

3 cloves garlic, minced

3 large carrots, diced

9 cup low-sodium beef broth

Ground black pepper, to taste

Direction:

1. Heat a large pot or Dutch oven over medium heat and add oil to it.

2. Once the oil is hot, stir the onion and garlic in, allowing them to cook for about three minutes, stirring often.

3. Stir carrots, beef, celery, and thyme into the pot. Brown the beef, breaking it into smaller chunks as you do so.

4. Once the beef is browned, add the broth, salt, pepper, and bay leaves to the pot, stirring completely. Cover the pot and bring to a boil.

5. Once boiling, reduce the heat to low and let simmer for 40 minutes.

6. Remove the pot from the heat and stir, adding the parsley and adjusting the seasoning to suit your taste. Remove the bay leaves and stir once more.

7. Serve hot!

Nutrition: Calories: 189 | Carbohydrates: 22g | Fat: 4g | Protein: 16g | Sugar: 3g

22. Instant Pot Chicken

Preparation Time: 5 min.

Cooking Time: 20 min.

Servings: 6

Ingredients: 1 cup water - 1 tsp. rosemary, chopped

1 medium lemon, sliced - 2 cloves garlic, minced

2 lb. chicken thighs, boneless & skinless

2 tbsps. extra virgin olive oil - Sea salt & pepper, to taste

Direction:

1.   Combine all ingredients in a medium mixing bowl, incorporate fully and cover.

2.   Plug in your Instant Pot and select the Sauté setting. Drizzle a little extra olive oil into the bottom of it to prevent sticking.

3.   Once the pot is hot, place the thighs in one even layer on the bottom of the Instant Pot and allow to cook until a golden crust is formed on the chick (about four to five minutes, then flip and allow the other side to cook as well.

4.   Pull the thighs out of the pot and use the water to deglaze the bottom of the pot, scraping lightly with your spatula or spoon as you stir the water around the pot. Place the chicken into the pot (on top of the trivet insert if you have one, but no problem if you don't) and place the lid on top. Cook at high pressure for five minutes to cook the chicken the rest of the way through. Release the pressure and remove the chicken from the pot. Serve hot with your favorite sides!

Nutrition: Calories: 223 | Carbohydrates: 0g | Fat: 11g | Protein: 30g | Sugar: 0g

23. Shrimp Salad

Preparation Time: 15 min.

Cooking Time: 0 min.

Servings: 8

Ingredients:

1/3 English cucumber, diced

¾ cup plain yogurt

1 lb. shrimp, cooked & chopped

1 tbsp. Dijon mustard

1 tsp. garlic powder

2 tbsps. mayo

3 medium stalks celery, diced

Sea salt & pepper, to taste

Direction

1.   In a large mixing bowl, combine all ingredients and stir to combine thoroughly.

2.   Cover and chill for at least 15 minutes before serving.

3.   Serve chilled!

Nutrition: Calories: 112 | Carbohydrates: 4g | Fat: 5g | Protein: 14g | Sugar: 3g

24. Broccoli Salad

Preparation Time: 20 min.

Cooking Time: 5 min.

Servings: 6

Ingredients:

½ cup dried cranberries, unsweetened

½ cup pecans, chopped

½ cup sunflower seeds

1 ½ tbsps. onion powder

1 cup plain yogurt

1 lb. broccoli, chopped

1 small bell pepper, diced

1 tbsp. apple cider vinegar

Red pepper flakes, to taste

Sea salt & pepper, to taste

Direction:

1.   In a large mixing bowl, combine all ingredients and stir to combine thoroughly.

2.   Cover and chill for at least 15 minutes before serving.

3.   Serve chilled!

Nutrition: Calories: 234 | Carbohydrates: 20g | Fat: 13g | Protein: 9g | Sugar: 9g

25. Southwest Chicken Salad

Preparation Time: 15 min.

Cooking Time: 15 min.

Servings: 8

Ingredients:

¼ cup extra virgin olive oil

¼ cup red onion, finely chopped

1 cup corn, drained

1 can low-sodium black beans, rinsed & drained

1 jalapeño, seeded & minced

1 tsp. chili powder

1 tsp. cumin

1 tsp. garlic powder

1 tsp. onion powder

2 bell peppers, diced

2 large limes, juiced

2 lb. chicken thighs, cooked and diced

2 tbsps. cilantro, finely chopped

3 cups quinoa, cooked to package instructions (still hot)

Sea salt & black pepper, to taste

Direction:

1.   In a small bowl, combine lime juice, chili powder, onion powder, garlic powder, cumin, and cilantro. Mix thoroughly and set aside.

2.   In a large mixing bowl, combine all other ingredients and toss until thoroughly combined.

3.   Drizzle seasoning mixture over the salad and toss to coat completely.

4.   Cover and chill for at least 30 minutes.

5.   Serve chilled!

Nutrition: Calories: 217 | Carbohydrates: 30g | Fat: 9g | Protein: 7g | Sugar: 2g

CHAPTER 19:

Frequently Asked Question About Intermittent Fasting

Is Intermittent Fasting Difficult To Adhere To?

It could be difficult for some people. You may experience difficulties and challenges, especially if you are still a beginner and your body even adjust and adapts to the new routine and food intake pattern. Once your body adapts, you will find the eating pattern more manageable and more comfortable to follow.

The central premise is being more aware of when and what you should eat. With such awareness, you will know precisely the boundaries and limitations you have to keep in mind. It would also be best to pair this approach with daily exercise and make healthy food choices, like fruits, beans, veggies, healthy fats, lean proteins, and lentils.

Avoiding too much sugar and sodium is a must, also. Once your body adapts to these new guidelines, adhering to IF will no longer be that challenging.

What Is the Recommended Number Of Hours/Days For Fasting?

In most cases, followers of the IF approach set their fasting window to up to 16 hours daily. Most follow this routine as it is a bit easy to adapt and adhere to. You can do it just by skipping breakfast after you ate your last meal the other day. If you can, you may also practice the IF pattern, which requires you to go without food for 24 hours straight twice every week.

Do I Still Need to Count Calories?

The answer to this will depend on the goals you want to achieve while practicing IF. It is unnecessary in some cases, but if your goal is to lose weight, you may want to monitor your calorie intake still.

Also, if you plan to cut out on snacks before sleeping or go without eating for an extended period, then you will notice your calorie count declining naturally. Another thing to note is that taking in foods that are mostly plant-based will also naturally lower your calorie intake.

Should Women Do IF Differently?

In most cases, men and women tend to respond differently to the IF protocol. Most women also agree that they tend to achieve better results by widening their eating window a bit. For instance, when trying to follow the 16/8 IF plan, some women noticed that they get better results after they modified the approach, increasing the number of eating hours to 10 and reducing the fasting hours to 14.

A wise piece of advice is to experiment and find out which one works for you. Observe the signals and cues sent by your body. Determine how it reacts to a specific IF pattern, too. Make sure to stick to an approach that seems to stimulate positive and favorable responses from your body.

Is It Safe for Pregnant or Breastfeeding Women to Fast?

Intermittent fasting is not highly recommended for pregnant women. It is mainly because your focus during pregnancy should be to supply your body with nutrients that can support your health and the growth and development of your baby. You need to eat highly nutritious foods that will help develop and build your baby's body and brain.

Also, take note that there are pregnant women who have a hard time having enough iron stores. If you do not eat the required foods every day, it might lead to iron deficiency, which is essential for your baby. Despite that, there is still no rule that bans pregnant women from practicing IF.

If you are one of those who have already practiced it and your health is at its best, then following IF is most likely safe for you. Just make sure that you only do it after receiving consent from your doctor. Also, it would be best to shorten the fasting period. If you are used to doing it for 24 hours or more, avoid doing it while pregnant. You should fast for at most 14 to 16 hours only.

If you are breastfeeding, long fasting periods also need to be avoided. It is because of the constant need of your baby for nutritious milk. Fasting may significantly impact breast milk quality and production, so you have to be extra careful. A wise piece of advice is to avoid fasting for more than 12 to 14 hours if you are breastfeeding to ensure that milk production will not be interrupted.

Make sure to observe yourself and the body, too. If you notice that your milk supply suddenly dries up and you suspect it is because of IF, then stop fasting right away. Try to eat more regularly to find out if doing so resolves the issue. If you notice fasting extensively hampering your milk production, then maybe it is time to stop it for a while and just continue once you already stop breastfeeding.

Can I Still Work Out Even If I Am Doing IF?

Of course, you can. If your fasting period is 24 hours or more, you may want to schedule your workouts during your non-fasting days to ensure that you have more energy to complete the sessions. You can also see other women working out even during their fasting periods, especially if their fasting takes less than 24 hours.

It is because they notice how effective exercising during a fast is in building lean muscle mass. In general, you should schedule your exercise based on how your body feels and the workout habits you are used to.

CHAPTER 20:

Create Your Plan

- Step One - Create a Monthly Calendar

On a calendar, highlight the days you wish to fast, depending on the type of fast you have committed yourself to. Record a start and end time on your fasting days, so you know how you plan to begin and finish in the days leading up to your fast day.

Tick off your days; this will keep you motivated and on track!

- Step Two - Record Your Findings

Create a journal for your fasting journey. One or two days before the time, undertake to do your measurements. Weigh yourself first thing in the morning, after you have gone to the restroom, and before breakfast. Also, do not weigh yourself wearing heavy items as they may affect the outcome of the scale.

Measure your height as this figure is related to your BMI (body mass index) result.

Record the measurements around your hips and stomach area; if you wish, you can also measure your upper thighs and arms.

Please take a photo of yourself and place it into the journal, too; this is not to discourage you but to keep you focused on why you began this journey.

Jot down all of these findings and update them weekly in the journal.

A journal is also the perfect way to express how you are feeling and, of course, what you are most thankful for. A journal is an important way to track not just the physical aspects of the diet but also its mental aspects. Never undertake to doubt yourself; your journal should be a safe space for you to congratulate and to motivate yourself. Leave all the negative thoughts at the door!

- Step Three - Plan Your Meals

The easiest way to stick to any eating program is to plan your meals; 500 calorie meals tend to be simple and easy to create, but there are also many other more complex recipes for those who wish to spice things up. Who knows, perhaps you stumble across a meal you wish to eat outside of your fasting days. It is advised that you prepare your meals the day before your fast days; doing this helps you stay committed to the fast and limits food wastage.

Initially, and in the first few weeks, it is suggested that you keep your meal preparation and recipes simple so as not to overcomplicate the whole process. This also allows you to get used to counting your calories and knowing which foods work to keep you fuller versus those that left you feeling hungrier earlier than later.

Be sure to include your meal plan in your journal and on your calendar.

- Step Four - Reward Yourself

On the days where you may return to normal eating, it is essential to reward yourself. A small reward goes a long way in reminding yourself and your brain that what you are doing has merit and that it should be noticed.

A reward should cater to one of our primal needs; these needs include:

Self-actualization

Safety needs

Social needs

Esteem needs

Physiological needs such as food, water, air, clothing, and shelter.

Have a block of chocolate or buy yourself a new item of clothing to do anything that makes your heart happy!

- Step Five — Curb Hunger Pains

Initially, you will feel more discomfort when hungry, but these feelings will pass. If you do find yourself craving something, sip on black tea or coffee to help you through your day. Coffee is known to alleviate the feelings of being hungry; if you must add sweetener, do so at your discretion. Know that some sweeteners can cause the opposite effect and make you feel hungry.

- Step Six - Stay busy

Keeping busy means that the mind does not have time to dwell on your current state of affairs, especially if you find yourself reaching for a snack bar or cookie.

It is also wise to be implementing some sort of physical activity, even on your fasting days. A 20-minute walk before ending your fasting period will do wonders to help you reach the final stages of the fasting period.

- Step Seven - Practice Mindful Eating

As mentioned, we are inclined to eat for all sorts of reasons; happy, sad, it does not matter. The problem is that these feelings related to food become habitual, so we aren't starving, but because we feel good or even off, we seek to tuck into something delicious.

The art of eating mindfully is not to allow these habits to master your life. The concept is simple: teach yourself to look at something, for instance, a piece of cake, and think, "Do I need it or do I want it for other reasons?" You could decide to have a bite or two and leave the rest, but you may be less inclined to eat the whole slice (or whole cake) if you think mindfully about it.

The art of mindful eating is to revel in the food placed before you. Pay attention to colors, textures, and tastes. Savor each bite, even when eating an apple.

Your brain gradually begins to rewire itself when it comes to food and when it needs or wants something.

Practice mindful eating by:

Only eat when your body signals you to do so, when your stomach growls or if you feel faint, or if your energy levels are low.

Pay attention to what is both healthy and unhealthy for us.

Consider the environmental impact our food choices make.

Every time you take a bite of your meal, set your cutlery down.

• Step Eight - Practice Portion Control

Controlling portion sizes can be difficult for most; society has also regulated us to what we think is the size of an average portion should be. We have access to supersizing meals too, which does not help those struggling in the weight department. In 1961, Americans consumed 2,880 calories per day; by 2017, they consumed 3,600 calories, which is a 34% increase and an unhealthy one at that.

To help you navigate how to portion your food better, consider trying the following: when dishing up your food, try the following trick. Half of your plate should consist of healthy fruits and vegetables, one quarter should be made up of your starches such as potatoes, rice, or pasta, and the remaining quarter should be made up of lean meats or seafood.

Alternatively, try the following:

Dish up onto a smaller plate or into a smaller bowl.

Say no to upsizing a meal if offered.

Buy the smaller version of the product if available or divide the servings equally into packets. Eat half a meal at the restaurant and take the remaining half to enjoy the following day instead.

Go to bed early; it will stop any after-dinner eating.

- Step Nine - Get Tech Savvy

Modern-day society has plenty to offer us in terms of the apps we can use to help determine the steps we take, the calories we burn, the calories found in our foods, research, information, and motivation for lifestyle changes, especially diets and exercise. The list is endless. There are many apps on the market currently that can help you track your progress in fasting. The best intermittent fasting apps currently (at the time of writing), and in no particular order, are:

Zero

Fast Habit

Body Fast

Fasting

Vora

Ate Food Diary

CHAPTER 21:

The Importance of Lifestyle

Once you get started with intermittent fasting, you will soon notice a natural tendency towards a more generally healthy lifestyle. This is a quite common virtuous circle: you start with a single healthy choice; this makes you feel better, feeling better gives you the energy to go on with more nutritious options, in a snowball effect of wellness.

You will naturally know and feel what healthy changes you'll need to put into your life, and this will probably not only concern your body's health but mind and spirit. For instance, once I kept experiencing an increase in clarity, I naturally felt the desire to read more books and scheduled a daily "me-time" of 45 minutes, just me and my book, door closed and phone off.

So, now we will look at some aspects you should consider as a general lifestyle background for your intermittent fasting path. Still, this is just some advice, please listen to yourself and be ready to embrace your body, mind, and spirit suggestions.

Moderate, if you don't want to get rid of, alcohol.

Intermittent fasting has shown to diminish inflammation in your body.

In any case, alcohol may aggravate inflammation, limiting the benefits of this diet.

Chronic inflammation may advance different diseases, for example, heart disease, type 2 diabetes, and certain malignancies.

Research shows that inflammation from excessive drinking may prompt intestinal disorder, bacterial overgrowth, and anomalies in intestinal microorganisms.

High alcohol intake can likewise strain your liver, diminishing its capacity to sift through possibly damaging elements.

Together, these consequences for your intestine and liver may advance inflammation throughout your body, which can cause organ harm over time. Over the top alcohol intake can cause far-reaching inflammation in your body, slowing if not stopping the effects of intermittent fasting and conceivably prompting infections.

Also, consider that drinking alcohol can break your fast.

During a fast, you should avoid all foods and drinks for a certain amount of time.

In particular, intermittent fasting is intended to advance hormonal and physical changes —, for example, fat consumption and cell repair— that may benefit your health.

As alcohol contains calories, any amount of it during a fasting period will break your fast. Apart from that, it is perfectly acceptable to drink in moderation during your eating periods.

During fasting periods, your body starts cell repair processes like autophagy, in which old, harmed proteins are expelled from cells to produce more effective, healthier cells. This process may diminish your danger of malignancy, distances the issues of aging effects, and at any rate, somewhat clarifies why calorie limitation has been shown to expand life expectancy.

Ongoing animal studies showing that constant alcohol intake may hinder autophagy in the liver and fat tissue.

Picking better alcohol choices

As alcohol breaks your fast whenever expended during a fasting period, it is recommended to just drinking during your planned eating periods. You should likewise hold your intake under tight restraints. Moderate alcohol consumption is characterized as close to one drink a day for women and close to two a day for men.

While intermittent fasting does not have exacting standards for food and drink intake, some alcohol habits are healthier than others are and more averse to hinder your dietary routine.

To restrict your sugar and calorie intake, avoid cocktails and prefer wines. During intermittent fasting, it is ideal for drinking alcohol moderately and only during your eating windows.

The Unhindered Eating Trap

Anyone who has ever changed their diet to get a health benefit or a healthy weight realizes that you begin to desire foods recommended not to eat. A study published in 2017 affirmed that an increased drive to eat is a critical factor during a weight loss journey.

Nevertheless, this test is explicitly restricted to an intermittent fasting plan. Food limitation happens during certain restricted hours, and on the non-fasting hours or days of the program, you can, for the most part, eat anything you desire.

Keeping on with unhealthy foods may not be the healthiest way to pick up benefits from intermittent fasting; however, removing them during specific days restricts your overall intake and may, in the end, give benefits anyway.

Don't stop working out

Or start doing it if you didn't.

You don't need to be an athlete, but you can't afford a sedentary lifestyle. Some people may think that since they are fasting, they should save energy and rest a lot. Well, that's not exactly like this. You should exercise as much as you can (that could be a little for you, but still), just taking some care.

You should choose whether you would want to work out while fasting or after having eaten. On the chance that you stick to the early afternoon to 8 p.m. eating plan, this mainly comes down to whether you usually work out in the first part of the day or the evening. Remember that you can change your timetable to your necessities. If you want to work out toward the beginning of the day after eating, you can change your fasting and eating periods to do it.

Training During Fasting

Training in a fasted state requires a few supplements to keep your body in an anabolic state. The body utilizes amino acids for energy if you are training without a pre-exercise meal. Your supplements for fast ought to include glutamine and branched-chain amino acid (BCAA) supplements.

Following the early afternoon to 8 p.m. feeding plan, you fast from 8 p.m. until around noon. So, take your glutamine and BCAA enhancements, and then do your workout. Depending on how long your training will last, this will set your post-exercise meal around the early afternoon.

What number of meals you decide to have during your starting period is up to you; however, remember that eating less as often as possible can hold your yearning within proper limits and support your body's capacity to build muscle?

Training During Feeding Period

On the chance that you like to work out after eating, you can plan your exercise to fall in the afternoon (early around 1 p.m., or toward the evening, around 5 p.m.). If your workout session is, for the most part, in the late afternoon, have your pre-training meal around the early afternoon, work out, and afterward have your other meals.

For an evening session, have your first meal around early afternoon and your pre-exercise meal around 4 p.m. If you may want to have a post-training meal one hour after working out, you can do that, too.

Adjusting Your Calorie Intake

The main principles about intermittent fasting include a few directions of when and how to get your calories and macronutrients.

If you train while fasting, your BCAA supplement's calorie check should be calculated toward your complete calories of the day, even though it does not end your fasting period. People on intermittent fasting plans usually distribute fifty calories for their fasting period to consider things like supplements or refreshments. This implies you can, in any case, take cream and sugar in your espresso or tea, regardless of whether or not it is during your fasting period.

In case you eat a pre-training meal, it is preferable to keep it light. Your meal should include a protein source like poultry or fish and some carbs, for a total amount of 400-500 calories. This will give you the protein and complex starches that are often suggested for pre-exercise meals. If you do eat a pre-exercise meal, the BCAA supplements prescribed for fasting exercises are most likely redundant, but you might need to take them in any case, since having an overflow of BCAAs may now be helpful anyway.

Your post-training meal is the best time to take a large portion of your sugars and calories. About a big part of your total calories for the day ought to be eaten during your post-training meal.

Conclusion

If you are a woman over 50, intermittent fasting may be beneficial to you. However, it is not a cure-all. You need to consult your doctor before embarking on any kind of fast. Intermittent fasting is not recommended for women with a history of breast cancer, diabetes, or liver disease. Most women over 50 who try intermittent fasting report that they feel better throughout the day. This reinforces the idea that fasts can be part of our lives as we age, but a doctor must first be consulted before attempting one.

Several fasts can improve your health. While long-duration fasts can get very difficult, some short-duration fasts can be just as effective at improving your health. In general, it is essential to scale back long fasts if you have trouble with them. If you want to experiment with shorter duration fasts, try eating less and sleeping more for two days, and then eating normally the next two days. Fasting can be beneficial when used in a short duration cycle.

There is no specific time frame that should be used for intermittent fasting when trying to improve health because it all depends on the individual's circumstances and goals for the fast. For some people, intermittent fasting or longer-duration fasts are useful if they are trying to lose weight, while others use them to manage their diabetes or heart disease. Intermittent fasting is perfect for women over 50. It allows women to reap the benefits of moderate-length fasts without giving their bodies time to adapt to stress from food deprivation. Intermittent fasting can also help women who have trouble sleeping during long fasts since it does not require as much sleep time every night. Intermittent fasting allows people to have more time between meals, enabling them to avoid snacking, which can lead to gaining weight if eaten frequently while fasting.

Intermittent fasting is a popular weight-loss technique that has been making headlines lately. It involves limiting eating to a specific window of time each day and then allowing yourself to eat normally for the remainder of the day.

Intermittent fasting is not a diet but rather a way to increase your metabolism and lose weight. It works by resetting your body's clock to burn fat at a higher rate and increase your metabolic rate (the rate at which your body uses energy and processes toxins).

The best way to start intermittent fasting is by establishing reliable eating windows or time frames during which you allow yourself to eat normally. This gives your body time to switch from being in "fasting" mode, burning fat at a higher rate, to the "fed" way, where it burns sugar and carbs instead. Your weight loss will begin after you've achieved this goal.

However, if you find that you can't stop eating after a few hours despite having set an eating window for yourself, you may be suffering from intermittent fasting for women over 50.

Prone to heartburn and indigestion, women over 50 seem to suffer from these maladies frequently. Here are some things you can try to avoid this type of discomfort.

The most effective way to avoid heartburn and indigestion is to eat when your stomach is empty. You must eat slowly and chew your food thoroughly. If you have trouble with chewing, have a glass of water nearby so you can take small sips while you're eating. Sipping will help keep your food moving through the digestive system.

If you are eating with other people, everyone must sit down at the table simultaneously. Try to avoid eating in front of a television or a computer monitor while seated on the couch or your bed. People who eat in these ways tend to eat less than those who sit down at the table and talk with others around them at the table.

If you are having heartburn problems or indigestion, ask your doctor about prescription meds for heartburn or indigestion. These drugs are much better than over-the-counter products that can cause more harm than good. Occasional fasts are another option you may want to consider if you have frequent problems with heartburn and indigestion. However, if you do fast every day, make sure that you don't skip meals altogether because this can lead to health complications such as hypoglycemia or low blood sugar.